The Effective Management of Cancer Pain

The Effective Management of Cancer Pain

Edited by

Richard Hillier MD FRCP
*Chairman, Association for Palliative Medicine, and Consultant in Palliative Medicine,
Southampton University Hospitals NHS Trust, Southampton*

Ilora Finlay FRCGP FRCP
*Professor of Palliative Medicine and Consultant Physician, University of Wales College of
Medicine, Cardiff, and Director, Marie Curie Holme Tower, Penarth, Wales*

John Welsh BSc FRCP
*Professor in the Dr Olav Kerr Chair of Palliative Medicine,
Glasgow University, Glasgow, Scotland*

Andrew Miles MSc MPhil PhD
*UeL Professor of Health Services Research & UK Key Advances Series Organiser
at St Bartholomew's Hospital, London*

UeL University Centre for
Health Services Research

AESCULAPIUS MEDICAL PRESS
LONDON SAN FRANCISCO SYDNEY

The Association for
Palliative Medicine of
Great Britain and Ireland

Published by

Aesculapius Medical Press (London, San Francisco, Sydney)
UEL University Centre for Health Services Research
St Bartholomew's Hospital
London
EC1A 7BE

British Library Cataloguing in Publication Data

A catalogue record for this book is available from the British Library

ISBN 1 903044 05 7

While the advice and information in this book are believed to be true and accurate at the
time of going to press, neither the authors nor the publishers nor the sponsoring institutions
can accept any legal responsibility or liability for any errors or omissions that may be made.
In particular (but without limiting the generality of the preceding disclaimer) every effort has
been made to check drug usages; however, it is possible that errors have been missed.
Furthermore, dosage schedules are constantly being revised and new side-effects recognised.
For these reasons, the reader is strongly urged to consult the drug companies' printed
instructions before administering any of the drugs recommended in this book.

Further copies of this volume are available from:

Claudio Melchiorri
Research Dissemination Fellow
UEL Centre for Health Services Research
St Bartholomew's Hospital
London EC1A 7BE

Fax: 0171 601 7085
e-mail: c.melchiorri@mds.qmw.ac.uk

Typeset, printed and bound in Britain by
Peter Powell Origination & Print Limited

Contents

Contributors

Graeme Bailie MB FRCS(I), Specialist Registrar in Orthopaedic Surgery, Belfast City Hospital/Northern Ireland Cancer Centre, Belfast, Northern Ireland

Stephen Barclay MA MB BCh MRCGP DipPallMed, General Practitioner, Health Services Research Training Fellow, and Honorary Consultant Physician in Palliative Medicine (Primary Care), General Practice and Primary Care Research Unit, Institute of Public Health, Cambridge

Jennifer Barraclough DM FRCP FRCPsych, Consultant in Psychological Medicine, Churchill Hospital, Oxford

Anthony Byrne MRCP(I), Marie Curie Consultant in Palliative Medicine, Velindre NHS Trust, Cardiff, Wales

P Declan Carey MB MCh FRCS(I), Consultant Surgical Oncologist/Clinical Leader Gastrointestinal Cancer, Belfast City Hospital/Northern Ireland Cancer Centre, and Honorary Senior Lecturer in Surgery, Queens University, Belfast, Northern Ireland

Bernadette A Corcoran MB MRCP(I), Macmillan Consultant in Palliative Care, Belfast City Hospital/Northern Ireland Cancer Centre, and Belvoir Park Regional Oncology Centre, Belfast, Northern Ireland

Ian AC Douglas MB ChB MRCGP, Specialist Registrar in Palliative Medicine, Yorkshire Deanery

Polly M Edmonds MBBS MRCP, Clinical Senior Lecturer, Department of Palliative Care and Policy, King's College London, and St Christopher's Hospice, London

Michael Frost BSc MSc DClinPsy AFBPsS, Consultant Clinical Psychologist, Pain Management Centre, Bronllys Hospital, Brecon, Wales

Geoffrey Hanks MB FRCP FRCPE FFPM, Macmillan Professor of Palliative Medicine, University of Bristol, Bristol Oncology Centre, Bristol

Colette Hawkins BSc MB MRCP, Macmillan Lecturer in Palliative Medicine, University of Bristol, Bristol Oncology Centre, Bristol

Irene J Higginson BMedSci BMBS FFPHM PhD, Professor of Palliative Care and Policy, King's College London, and St Christopher's Hospice, London

Richard Hillier MD FRCP, Chairman, Association for Palliative Medicine, and Consultant in Palliative Medicine, Countess Mountbatten House, Southampton University Hospitals NHS Trust, Southampton

Allan T Irvine MRCP FRCR, Honorary Senior Lecturer, UMDS, Consultant Radiologist, Department of Radiology, St Thomas' Hospital, London

Rosemary F Lennard MBChB FRCP PhD, Consultant in Palliative Medicine, Bradford

Bee Wee MB BCh(U.Dubl.) MCGP(I), Senior Lecturer and Consultant in Palliative Medicine, Countess Mountbatten House, Southampton University Hospitals NHS Trust, Southampton

Linda Wilson MB ChB MRCGP, Specialist Registrar in Palliative Medicine, Yorkshire Deanery

Preface

Cancer pain is common and widely feared. The advent of the World Health Organization analgesic ladder has provided doctors worldwide with the means to relieve up to 80 per cent of pain in patients with cancer. Yet the journals regularly report poor pain control in hospitals and in the community, in both the West and the developing world. The reasons for this are probably complex and are related to lack of knowledge and skills, myths about cancer pain and the effectiveness of existing treatments.

This volume presents a wide-angled approach to the effective management of cancer pain. It begins by examining the current literature on the efficacy both of current treatments and of our ability to assess effectiveness. Evidence-based management relies on two main themes. First, the systematic review of current trials and, second, professional judgement and clinical experience. These are discussed separately.

One of the key issues in delivering effective treatment is to make a thorough assessment of pain. A careful history must be taken to make an accurate diagnosis. The role of radiological investigation in the diagnosis of pain is considered in Chapter 4. However, with such a complex, multifactorial symptom as pain there are psychosocial, functional and spiritual issues to be evaluated which are as important as the pathology. These are examined in Chapter 5.

Since time immemorial, morphine has been considered the gold standard for cancer pain management. Is this still true or has the recent plethora of new drugs, or old drugs in different formulations, supplanted oral morphine? This is discussed in Chapter 6, while a similar analysis of non-steroidal anti-inflammatory drugs is covered in Chapter 7. No book on cancer pain management would be complete without a discussion of difficult pains. Chapter 8 looks at the issue of how pains vary with time and how little this has been addressed in the past. Though what might appear as a simple issue, this may have considerable implications for future practice and is little understood.

The surgical management of cancer pain is necessary in relatively few patients. However, it is crucial that, as part of an overall package of pain control, this is considered. When in doubt, ask. Finally, the book ends by focusing on patients where they spend most of their time, namely, at home. Despite an increasingly high quality of community care, effective pain management is still a problem, although recent work indicates that pain control at home may be better than in hospital.

In the current age, where doctors and health professionals are increasingly overwhelmed by clinical information, we have aimed to provide a fully current, fully referenced text which is as succinct as possible but as comprehensive as necessary. Consultants and specialist registrars in palliative medicine will find it of particular use as part of their continuing medical education and specialist training, and we advance it explicitly as an excellent tool for these purposes. We anticipate, however, that the book will prove of not inconsiderable use to other members of the palliative care team as a reference text, and to commissioners of health services as the basis for discussion and negotiation of health contracts with their practising colleagues.

In conclusion, we thank Napp Pharmaceuticals Ltd for the grant of educational sponsorship which helped organise a national symposium on cancer pain at the Royal College of Physicians, at which synopses of the constituent chapters of this book were presented.

Richard Hillier MD FRCP
Ilora Finlay FRCGP FRCP
John Welsh BSc FRCP
Andrew Miles MSc MPhil PhD

PART 1

Evidence and assessment

Chapter 1

Effectiveness and efficiency in the management of cancer pain: current dilemmas in clinical practice

Irene J Higginson and Polly M Edmonds

Introduction

Pain is one of the most common symptoms experienced by cancer patients. The last 20 years have seen great progress in the management of cancer pain. However, the significance of the symptom to patients and their families, its high prevalence and the complex nature of pain in cancer mean that effective clinical management is a continuing priority. This chapter analyses current dilemmas in determining effectiveness in the management of cancer pain and the implications of implementing research findings in clinical practice.

Effectiveness and efficiency as part of quality of care

Quality of health care has five components: effectiveness, efficacy, efficiency, humanity and equity. Effectiveness analyses whether a therapy works in general conditions, whereas efficacy analyses whether a therapy has been tested in ideal conditions, usually a randomised controlled trial. Efficiency assesses whether a therapy is good value for money, benefiting the maximum number of people for a given cost. Humanity assesses whether a therapy is considered as acceptable and humane by the people who need it. Equity is whether a therapy is equally received by all those people who need it. All of these components are important in assessing treatments in the management of cancer pain. In practical terms, efficacy is often determined first – with therapies being developed in laboratory conditions and then tested in very controlled conditions. The effectiveness of any treatment is altered by the humanity and the equity of delivery because it relates to how treatments work in the 'real world'. Throughout the world health care costs are often constrained and therefore efficiency – value for money – is often important.

Evidence-based practice seeks to integrate the best evidence from research studies, clinical experience and the individual wishes of patients and families. When developing evidence-based practice in the management of cancer pain, several dilemmas face us. First, there is the problem of pain assessment with wide variations in the prevalence of cancer pain. Second, much of the evidence about the effectiveness and efficacy of pain control is lacking. Third, there is a need in clinical practice to develop better monitoring systems so that more information about effectiveness can be collected. These issues are considered in turn.

Pain assessment

The prevalence of pain is often poorly understood and reported. The proportion of cancer patients with pain varies from study to study depending upon the stage of disease included, the detection, assessment and measurement of pain, and the interactions with other problems considered. It may also be different according to whether pain is investigated by a doctor, a nurse, in a research study, or in a clinical context. Those studies that have included patients with advanced or far advanced cancer have tended to examine patients in particular settings – such as oncology departments, cancer hospitals, or hospices (Table 1.1) (Higginson 1997; Hearn & Higginson 1999). In these groups of patients, depending upon the methods of the study, between 58 and 84 per cent of cancer patients were assessed as having pain.

The prevalence of pain for different types of cancer varies enormously, depending upon stage of disease and assessment (see Table 1.2). For example, different studies found that the prevalence of pain ranged from 40 to 89 per cent among patients with breast cancer and from 17 to 74 per cent among patients with lung cancer. Late-stage cancer is associated with more pain than earlier stages of disease, and this explains some of the variation. However, as a result of these variations, it can be difficult for individual clinicians to compare their practice with others and to interpret the relevance of some of their research findings to their own practice.

Evidence of the effectiveness of pain control

Much of the evidence about the effectiveness and efficiency of pain control is incomplete among patients with progressive illness. The clinician often must make decisions to treat based on small or observational studies and in some instances on case reports.

The WHO analgesic ladder

Between 1982 and 1984 an expert committee, convened by the World Health Organization (WHO) Cancer Pain Relief Programme, developed guidelines for managing cancer pain, with the aim of improving pain control in cancer patients worldwide. The final version of these guidelines (World Health Organization 1987) has as its core a three-step analgesic ladder based on pain severity, rather than aetiology, which can be implemented in any care setting. The guidelines suggest that patients with cancer pain receive regular oral analgesia. Step one of the ladder recommends the use of non-opioid analgesics (such as paracetamol) for mild-to-moderate pain; step two recommends opioids for moderate pain (such as dihydrocodeine); and step three recommends opioids for severe pain (such as morphine). Co-analgesics may be considered on any step of the ladder in addition to non-opioid or opioid analgesics.

Table 1.1 Prevalence of cancer pain in different settings

Stage	Setting for sample and reference	% with pain	n
Ambulatory patients	Cancer hospital (Portenoy et al. 1992)	33	326
All stages	Cancer hospital* (Foley 1979)	38	397
All stages	Cancer hospital (Daut & Cleeland 1982)	49	667
All stages	20 study review** (Bonica 1990)	53	4,346
All stages	Multicentre study (Hiraga et al. 1991)	33	35,683
All stages	Multicentre study (Cleeland et al. 1994)	67	1,308
All stages	Cancer hospital (Portenoy et al. 1994)	64	243
All stages	Multicentre study (Larue et al. 1995)	57	605
Advanced	Oncology department (Pannuti et al. 1979)	64	291
Advanced	Oncology outpatients (Trotter et al. 1981)	72	237
Advanced	Hospital team (Ellershaw et al. 1995)	74	125
Last year of life	Bereaved carers all settings (Addington-Hall 1993)	88	2,018
Far advanced	Hospice (Twycross 1974)	84	500
Far advanced	Cancer hospital* subanalysis of report above	60	39
Far advanced	Community (Higginson & Hearn 1997)	70	695
Advanced/terminal	32 study review** sub-analysis of report above data (e.g. adjusted to not include those studies given elsewhere in the table)	79	7,940

Source: Adapted from Higginson & Hearn (1997)

An initial, retrospective validation study on 292 patients completing all three steps of the ladder demonstrated a significant reduction in the mean pain score ($p < 0.01$) and a significant increase in hours of sleep ($p < 0.001$), with no reduction in performance status (Ventafridda et al. 1987). Zech et al. (1995) reported on a prospective evaluation of 2,118 patients receiving analgesics in accordance with the WHO ladder over 140,478 treatment days. Non-opioid analgesics were administered on 11 per cent of treatment days, opioids for moderate pain on 31 per cent and opioids for severe pain on 49 per cent of treatment days. Co-analgesics were used on 37 per cent of treatment days. A highly significant reduction in pain was documented within the first week ($p < 0.001$), and 76 per cent of treated patients achieved good pain relief. However, a systematic review highlighted some of the difficulties in interpreting the validation studies (Jadad & Browman 1995). Of eight studies identified for the review none had used control groups, two were retrospective, there was little information on the conditions under which the pain was assessed, the follow-up was variable, and three studies had high withdrawal rates. Analgesia was adequate in 69–100 per cent of patients analysed in the studies.

The lack of a control group in any of these studies does not mean that the ladder is ineffective, rather that the proportion of patients achieving adequate pain relief using the ladder may be overestimated. The great strength of the WHO ladder, however, lies in its simplicity and logical step-wise approach to managing pain.

Table 1.2 Prevalence of pain by primary tumour site (%)

Tumour site	Foley 1979	Daut & Cleeland* 1982	Greenwald et al. 1987	Simpson 1991	Portenoy et al. 1994	Donnelly et al. 1995	Larue et al. 1995	Vainio & Auvinen 1996	Higginson & Hearn 1997	No. of studies	Mean$ %	Range of %
Breast	52	64; 40		50	60	89	56	78	76	8	64	40–89
Lung	45		71	17			58	74	71	6	56	17–74
Prostate		75; 30	56		68	94		83		5	74	56–94
Genitourinary	70–75			88			58	90	74	5	77	58–90
Lymphoma	20			50			35	87	74	5	53	20–87
Colo-(rectal)	40	47; 40			62	79		79		4	65	40–79
Gastrointestinal				50–71			56		68	4	56	40–68
Cervix†		0; 35	56			87				3	59	33–87
Head and neck						91	67	83		3	80	67–91
Ovary		59; 39			67	71				3	61	46–71

* Metastatic disease; non-metastatic disease. NB: an overall percentage was determined for each cancer type from the original article, not given here

$ Calculated using the overall percentage values where necessary

† Cervix/cervix-vagina/uterine cervix

Source: Adapted from Higginson & Hearn (1999)

Over 15 years of clinical experience supports the premise that most cancer pain can be treated with analgesic drugs, and supports its continued use, both as a clinical and educational model for managing chronic pain.

Alternative opioid analgesics

While morphine remains the 'gold-standard' strong opioid for moderate-to-severe pain (see Chapter 6), in recent years several alternative strong opioids have become available in preparations tailored to patients with pain from malignant disease, such as hydromorphone and transdermal fentanyl. In the UK, oxycodone is due to be launched in immediate-release and controlled-release preparations in the near future. Side-effects are common with all opioid preparations, and whether unacceptable adverse effects occur before adequate analgesia is achieved depends on a complex interrelationship between patient, drug and pain-related factors. There is no evidence to suggest that any alternative opioid analgesics provide superior pain relief to morphine and little to suggest that the side-effect profile varies markedly; one study, however, has suggested that transdermal fentanyl is less constipating than oral morphine in equi-analgesics doses (Ahmedzai & Brooks 1997).

Opioid rotation

The term 'opioid rotation' is used to describe the switch from one opioid drug to another in order to minimise drug-related toxicity and improve analgesia. The factors underlying the concept of opioid rotation are complex and controversial (Twycross 1974; Fallon 1997a, 1997b), but an important factor may be incomplete cross-tolerance between different opioid drugs in terms of both analgesic efficacy and toxicity. In one centre 58 of 80 (73 per cent) patients undergoing opioid rotation for unacceptable side-effects were reported to have improvements in opioid-related toxicity associated with significant improvements in pain control, at doses significantly lower than that predicted to be equi-analgesic (De Stoutz et al. 1995). Several other studies have supported these observations, most commonly for patients with opioid-related cognitive impairment or hyperexcitability (Sjorgren et al. 1994; Maddocks et al. 1996; Hagen and Swanson 1998; Ashby et al. 1999). Controversy remains as to the optimal policy for managing opioid-related toxicity, and the frequency of opioid rotation varies markedly between centres, but in the UK it may be required in as few as 2–3 per cent of patients taking strong opioid analgesics (Hawley et al. 1997).

A pragmatic approach to patients who become confused or agitated while taking opioid analgesics could include the following:

- review the cause(s) of the pain;
- exclude and treat any potentially confounding factors, such as dehydration or hypercalcaemia;
- reduce the opioid dose;
- adjust the dose of, or introduce, co-analgesics.

If simple measures such as those described above do not improve the clinical situation, then substitution of one opioid analgesic for another may be appropriate; the choice of opioid will depend on the preparations available and prescriber's choice.

Use of co-analgesics

The WHO advocates the use of co-analgesics (adjuvant analgesics) to optimise pain control for patients on all three steps of the analgesic ladder. Examples of co-analgesics include tricyclic antidepressant drugs (TCADs), anticonvulsants, antiarrhythmics, muscle relaxants (e.g. benzodiazepines, baclofen), non-steroidal anti-inflammatory drugs (NSAIDs), corticosteroids and N-methyl D-aspartate (NMDA) receptor antagonists (e.g. ketamine). The co-analgesics that will be discussed further in this article are antidepressants, anticonvulsants and antiarrythmics. NSAIDs are covered in Chapter 7.

Antidepressants

There is good evidence that TCADs are analgesic in a variety of chronic pain syndromes, the mechanism of action probably involving inhibition of re-uptake of noradrenalin and serotonin in the spinal cord. A systematic review analysed data from 21 placebo-controlled treatments in 17 randomised controlled trials for patients with a variety of chronic pain syndromes, such as atypical facial pain, central pain and post-herpetic neuralgia (McQuay *et al.* 1996). The overall number needed to treat (NNT) for benefit (i.e. more than 50 per cent improvement in pain intensity/relief for one patient) was 2.9 (95 per cent confidence interval 2.4–3.7), the NNT for minor (expected) adverse effects was 3.7 (2.9–5.2) and for major adverse effects, necessitating withdrawal of the drug, 22 (13.5–58). There was no difference in efficacy or toxicity between the different TCADs studied, but the serotonin selective re-uptake inhibitors (SSRIs) appeared less effective analgesics.

It is less clear whether the evidence for the efficacy of TCADs in chronic pain is directly transferable to the cancer population. Neuropathic pain in cancer may occur as a direct result of nerve injury (compression or infiltration) caused by the cancer or from treatment, and frequently occurs as part of a mixed-pain syndrome. It may be more acute in onset than other chronic pain states, and may be more opioid-responsive than other chronic pain states (Fallon & Hanks 1993). There are several, largely uncontrolled, trials assessing the efficacy of TCADs in cancer-related pain, but only two placebo-controlled studies with small numbers of patients. In a placebo-controlled cross over study, 28 of 40 patients receiving imipramine 75 mg o.d. had improved pain, compared to 18 receiving placebo (p<0.06) (Fiorentino 1967). A placebo-controlled study of amitriptyline (median dose 50 mg/day) in 15 patients with post-mastectomy pain demonstrated more than 50 per cent reduction in pain intensity on a visual analogue scale in eight patients (53 per cent), and significant improvements in pain intensity and pain relief compared to placebo (p<0.05) (Eija *et al.* 1995).

There are, however, multiple unanswered questions relating to the use of TCADs in cancer pain: the optimal drug, starting dose, speed of dose titration and maximum dose for therapeutic benefit all remain to be determined.

Anticonvulsants

Anticonvulsants are widely used in the management of both chronic non-malignant pain and cancer-related pain. A systematic review of 20 randomised controlled trials of four anticonvulsants has been undertaken. The results for common pain syndromes are summarised in Table 1.3.

One controlled study of anticonvulsants in cancer pain has been identified (Yajnik *et al.* 1992). This parallel group study of four weeks' duration compared buprenorphine alone, phenytoin alone and buprenorphine and phenytoin in combination, with pain relief and pain intensity as the main outcome measures: 21/25 in the buprenorphine group, 18/25 in the phenytoin group and 22/25 combination patients achieved good or moderate pain relief. Adverse effects were less common in the phenytoin and combination groups.

There are also multiple unanswered questions regarding anticonvulsants in cancer pain, many of which are similar to those with TCADs. While they appear to be effective analgesics as a group in some chronic pain states, the anticonvulsants are a heterogeneous group of drugs with different mechanisms of action. Phenytoin and carbamazepine are sodium channel blockers; phenytoin also enhances gamma-aminobutyric acid (GABA) activity. Sodium valproate is a GABA agonist, but probably has multiple mechanisms of action, including effects on sodium and calcium channels. A number of newer anticonvulsant drugs have recently been promoted for the management of pain. Gabapentin may promote release of GABA, but its precise mechanism of action as an anticonvulsant and analgesic is unknown. Lamotrigine is thought to act by inhibiting glutamate release, but also has effects on sodium channels. In randomised placebo-controlled trials, gabapentin has been shown to have analgesic activity in patients with post-herpetic neuralgia (Rowbotham *et al.* 1998), and lamotrigine in patients with refractory trigeminal neuralgia (Zakrzewska *et al.* 1997). It is likely that as the mechanisms of these different drugs in chronic pain states become better understood, their role in the management of cancer pain will be more clearly defined. Controlled studies of both new and old anticonvulsants will be required to determine

Table 1.3 Systematic review of anticonvulsants for pain

	NNT for effectiveness	NNT for minor adverse effect	NNT for major adverse effect
Trigeminal neuralgia (3 studies)	2.6	3.4	24
Diabetic neuropathy (2 studies)	2.5	3.1	20
Migraine prophylaxis (3 studies)	1.6	2.4	39

NNT = number needed to treat

Source: McQuay *et al.* (1995)

their role more clearly, and in future it will no longer be possible to discuss the role of anticonvulsants in cancer pain as if they were a distinct group of drugs.

Antiarrhythmics

Systemically administered local anaesthetic-type drugs are sodium channel blockers that can also be used for the management of chronic pain, most commonly in palliative care after trials of antidepressants and/or anticonvulsants have failed. A systematic review identified 17 randomised controlled trials of local anaesthetics for chronic pain (McQuay 1997). There was good evidence to support the use of intravenous lignocaine and oral mexiletine for patients with peripheral nerve injury, where the reduction in pain intensity was of the order of 40–60 per cent and allodynia and dysaesthesia were alleviated. The evidence for efficacy in diabetic neuropathy and post-herpetic neuralgia was weaker. The review identified three studies of intravenous lignocaine in cancer-related pain (pain due to bone metastases; chemotherapy-induced polyneuropathy and radiation-induced plexopathy; and tumour infiltration). Lignocaine had no effect in any of these pain states. There are no controlled trials of the efficacy of oral agents (mexiletine or flecainide) in cancer-related pain.

Issues in measuring efficiency and costs

Whether therapies represent value for money is asked increasingly, as the pressure on health care budgets grows. Costs come in several categories: the cost of the drugs or treatments, the wider costs to health care (such as inpatient hospital days, community visits), the costs to other forms of care, such as social or voluntary services, and the costs to the patient and their family. Ideally, any evaluation would determine the outcomes in terms of relief of pain and suffering and reduced side-effects *versus* the costs. In cost-effectiveness analysis costs are compared for treatments aimed at patients with broadly similar problems (for example, reducing pain in advanced cancer patients). In cost-utility or cost-benefit analysis costs are compared for treatments intended for very different patients (such as to compare the benefits of treatments for diabetes and cancer). Cost-effectiveness analysis is the method most commonly used to compare treatments designed to control pain.

Clinicians often make simple comparisons of the costs of drugs to help to guide practice. The WHO guidance on essential drugs for cancer therapy recommends the use of cheap effective drugs for pain control, in addition to 17 relatively cheap and effective anticancer drugs (Sikora *et al.* 1999). Such comparisons are valuable in minimising costs. Evaluations of pain therapies rarely have assessed costs and when they have, the costs of only the hospital services, rather than wider aspects of care, have been included. More work is needed in this area.

A way forward: clinical monitoring systems

Data-collection is most problematic in late-stage cancer where patients find it difficult to record pain assessments. The initial assessment and recording of pain in studies, using a detailed body chart, is important. Repeated assessment, so that pain can be monitored over time, using some of the questionnaires and standardised measures in palliative care, is now possible (Hearn & Higginson 1997). Some of these measures, such as the new palliative outcome scale (Hearn & Higginson forthcoming), have been validated to use proxies, such as the carer or doctor or nurse, to record the assessment alongside the patient, thus allowing better assessment and monitoring even in advanced disease. Such monitoring will provide more information on the effectiveness of pain treatments in clinical practice.

A way forward: using the evidence

A further clinical issue is the interdependence of pain with other physical, emotional, social and spiritual issues. The management of cancer pain is based on a team approach, whose interventions are difficult to separate. When clinicians apply treatments shown elsewhere to benefit patients, they may need to provide all components of care to achieve similar results. Similarly, treatments which work in inpatient settings may not apply easily to home care, because of compliance or available facilities. Community-based studies of pain control are less common (Higginson & Hearn 1997).

When deciding to use clinical treatments, we would propose that a biological rationale, although useful, is insufficient alone. Equally, because of the lack of randomised controlled trials and the difficulty in conducting these in the palliative population, in addition to evidence from randomised trials, evidence from prospective and retrospective studies and clinical monitoring is also important. Instead, when selecting treatments the clinician could look for a combination of some of the following aspects of evidence:

- evidence of clinical effectiveness (randomised trials would be the highest-ranking evidence, but other studies would be important) in the group of patients undergoing treatment;
- evidence of clinical effectiveness in analogous groups of patients to those undergoing treatment (here randomised trials may be available);
- similarity of the 'team' or service setting in which the therapy was developed;
- biological rationale for the treatment;
- evidence of pharmacokinetic data to influence use (for example, a dose-response curve).

Any treatment will need to be tailored to the individual's needs and their response to it. Evidence-based practice encourages the discussion of treatment choices with patients and their families, and to achieve this clinicians must also be sufficiently trained in communication skills.

References

Addington-Hall JM (1993). *Regional study of the care for the dying. Feedback for district health authorities. Cancer deaths only.* Department of Epidemiology and Public Health, University College London, London.

Ahmedzai S & Brooks D (1997). Transdermal fentanyl versus oral morphine in cancer pain: preference, efficacy and quality of life. *Journal of Pain and Symptom Management* **13**, 254–61.

Ashby MA, Martin P & Jackson KA (1999). Opioid substitution to reduce adverse effects in cancer pain management. *Medical Journal Australia* **170**, 68–71.

Bonica JJ (1990). Cancer pain. In *The management of cancer pain* (ed. JJ Bonica), pp.400–60. Lea & Febiger, Philadelphia, USA.

Cleeland CS, Gonin R, Hatfield AK, Edmondson JH, Blum RH, Stewart JA & Pandya KJ (1994). Pain and its treatment in outpatients with metastatic cancer. *New England Journal of Medicine* **330**, 592–6.

Daut RL & Cleeland CS (1982). The prevalence and severity of pain in cancer. *Cancer* **50**, 1913–18.

De Stoutz ND, Bruera E & Suarez-Alazor M (1995). Opioid rotation for toxicity reduction in terminally ill patients. *Journal of Pain and Symptom Management* **10**, 378–84.

Eija K, Tiina T & Pertti J (1995). Amitriptyline effectively relieves neuropathic pain following treatment of breast cancer. *Pain* **64**, 293–302.

Ellershaw JE, Peat SJ & Boys LC (1995). Assessing the effectiveness of a hospital palliative care team. *Palliative Medicine* **9**, 145–52.

Fallon M (1997a). Opioid rotation: does it have a role. *Palliative Medicine* **12**, 60–1.

Fallon M (1997b). Opioid rotation: does it have a role? [Reply]. *Palliative Medicine* **12**, 61–2.

Fallon M & Hanks GWC (1993). Opioid resistant pain in cancer: sense or nonsense. *The Pain Clinic* **6**, 205–6.

Fiorentino G (1967). Sperimentazione controllata dell'imipramina come analgesico maggiore in oncologia. *Rivista Medica Trentina* **5**, 387–97.

Foley KM (1979). Pain syndromes in patients with cancer. In *Advances in pain research and therapy* (ed. JJ Bonica & V Ventafridda), pp.59–75. Raven Press, New York, USA.

Greenwald HP, Bonica JJ & Bergner M (1987). The prevalence of pain in four cancers. *Cancer* **60**, 2563–9.

Hagen N & Swanson R (1998). Strychnine-like multifocal myoclonus and seizures in extremely high-dose opioid administration: treatment strategies. *Journal of Pain and Symptom Management* **15**, 143–4.

Hawley P, Forbes K & Hanks GW (1997). Opioids, confusion and opioid rotation [Letter]. *Palliative Medicine* **12**, 63–64.

Hearn J & Higginson IJ (1997). Outcome measures for advanced cancer patients: a review of current measures and the development of a national core measure. *Palliative Medicine* **11**, 71–2.

Hearn J & Higginson IJ (1999). Epidemiology of pain: pain associated with cancer. In *Task force on epidemiology*. International Association for the Study of Pain, Seattle, USA.

Hearn J & Higginson IJ (forthcoming). Development and validation of a core outcome measure for palliative care – The Palliative Care Outcome Scale (The P.O.S.). *Quality in Healthcare* (in press).

Higginson IJ (1997). *Innovations in assessment: epidemiology and assessment of pain in advanced cancer*. International Association for the Study of Pain, Seattle, USA.

Higginson IJ & Hearn J (1997). A multicentre evaluation of cancer pain control by palliative care teams. *Journal of Pain and Symptom Management* **14**, 29–35.

Hiraga K, Mizuguchi T & Takeda F (1991). The incidence of cancer pain and improvement of pain management in Japan. *Postgraduate Medicine Journal* **67**, S14–25.

Jadad AR & Browman GP (1995). The WHO analgesic ladder for cancer pain management. Stepping up the quality of its evaluation. *Journal of the American Medical Association* **274**, 1870–3.

Larue F, Colleau SM, Brasseur L & Cleeland CS (1995). Multicentre study of cancer pain and its treatment in France. *British Journal of General Practice* **310**, 1034–7.

McQuay HJ (1997). Systematic local anaesthetic type drugs in chronic pain. *Health Technology Assessment* **1**, 85–90.

McQuay H, Carroll D, Jadad AR, Witten P & Moore A (1995). Anticonvulsant drugs for management of pain: a systematic review. *BMJ* **311**, 1047–52.

McQuay HJ, Tramer M, Nye BA, Carroll D, Wiffen PJ & Moore RA (1996). A systematic review of antidepressants in neuropathic pain. *Pain* **68**, 217–27.

Maddocks I, Somogyi A, Abbott F, Hayball P & Parker D (1996). Attenuation of morphine-induced delirium in palliative care by substitution with infusion of oxycodone. *Journal of Pain and Symptom Management* **12**, 182–9.

Pannuti E, Rossi AP & Marraro D (1979). Natural history of cancer pain. In *The continuing care of terminal patients* (ed. RG Twycross & V Ventafridda), pp.75–89. Pergamon, New York, USA.

Portenoy RK, Miransky J, Tahler R, Hornung J, Bianchi C, Cibas-Kong I, Feldhamer E, Lewis F, Matamoros I, Sugar MZ, Olivieri AP, Kemeny NE & Foley KM (1992). Pain in ambulatory patients with lung or colon cancer: prevalence, characteristics, and effect. *Cancer* **70**, 1616–24.

Portenoy RK, Thaler HT, Kornblith AB, Lepore JM, Friedlander-Klar H, Coyle N, Smart-Curley T, Kemeny NE, Norton L, Hoskins W & Scher H (1994). Symptom prevalence, characteristics and distress in a cancer population. *Quality of Life Research* **3**, 183–9.

Rowbotham M, Harden N, Stacey B, Bernstein P & Magnus-Miller L (1998). Gabapentin for the treatment of postherpetic neuralgia: a randomised controlled trial. *Journal of the American Medical Association* **280**, 1837–42.

Sikora K, Advani S, Koroltchouk V, Magrath I, Levy L, Pinedo H, Schwartsemann G, Tattersall M & Yan S (1999). Essential drugs for cancer therapy: a World Health Organization consultation. *Annals of Oncology* **10**, 385–90.

Simpson M (1991). The use of research to facilitate the creation of a hospital palliative care team. *Palliative Medicine* **5**, 122–9.

Sjorgren P, Jensen NH & Jensen TS (1994). Disappearance of morphine-induced hyperalgesia after discontinuing or substituting morphine with other opioid agonists. *Pain* **59**, 313–16.

Trotter JM, Scott R, Macbeth FR, McVie JG & Calman KC (1981). Problems of oncology outpatients: role of the liaison health visitor. *British Medical Journal of Clinical Research Education* **282**, 122–4.

Twycross RG (1974). Clinical experience with diamorphine in advanced malignant disease. *International Journal of Clinical Pharmacology* **67**, 184–98.

Vainio A & Auvinen A (1996). Prevalence of symptoms among patients with advanced cancer: an international collaborative study. Symptom Prevalence Group. *J Pain Symptom Management* **12**, 3–10.

Ventafridda V, Tamburini M, Caraceni A, De Conno F & Naldi F (1987). A validation study of the WHO method for cancer pain relief. *Cancer* **59**, 850–6.

World Health Organization (1987). *Cancer pain relief.* WHO, Geneva, Switzerland.

Yajnik S, Singh GP, Singh G & Kumar M (1992). Phenytoin as a coanalgesic in cancer pain. *Journal of Pain and Symptom Management* **7**, 209–13.

Zakrzewska JM, Chaudhry Z, Nurmikko TJ, Patton DW & Mullens EL (1997). Lamotrigine in refractory trigeminal neuralgia: results from a double blind placebo controlled crossover trial. *Pain* **73**, 23–30.

Zech DFJ, Grond S, Lynch J, Hertel D & Lehmann KA (1995). Validation of the WHO guidelines for cancer pain relief: a 10-year prospective study. *Pain* **63**, 65–76.

Chapter 2

The role of systematic overviews of the research literature in identifying clinical evidence for pain management

Michael Frost

Introduction

Evidence-based medicine has been defined by Sackett *et al.* (1996) as 'the conscientious, explicit, and judicious use of current best evidence in making decisions about the care of the individual patient'. Since the practical demands of caring for patients leave little time for clinicians to keep up with current evidence, the task of deciding which is the best has traditionally devolved on academic reviewers and the opinion of experts. Neither can be completely trusted. As Trisha Greenhalgh (1997) has pointed out, a literature review often tends towards the journalistic with the author selecting the papers that support a personal view and leaving out those that cause embarrassment. This is unfortunate, but at least the bias is easily recognised, which is not always the case with an expert opinion. In 1996, for example, a National Institute of Health assessment panel concluded, without referencing a single primary source, that the evidence for the effectiveness of several behavioural and relaxation interventions in the treatment of chronic pain was 'relatively good' (NIH Technology Assessment Panel 1996). It is not surprising that reports by expert committees rank equal bottom with opinions of respected authorities in McQuay & Moore's (1998) league table for 'strength of efficacy' evidence.

Top of the league comes strong evidence from at least one systematic review of multiple, well-designed randomised controlled trials (RCTs). The usefulness of a systematic review, however, depends upon the reviewer posing a clearly focused clinical question and finding, if not all, most of the relevant high-quality trials, and in sufficient numbers to answer the question. This is a particular difficulty in reviewing strategies for cancer pain management. There are few good studies to be found, tempting reviewers to ask too broad a question. For example, Sindhu (1996) attempted to determine the effectiveness of non-pharmacological nursing interventions for the management of pain. A literature search yielded 3,166 abstracts, only 49 of which were considered to be of sufficient quality to be included in a systematic review. With the emphasis on quality up front, content took the back seat, and interventions as diverse as surgical collars, biofeedback and music were included in the meta-analysis. Naturally, the breadth of the question and the all-inclusive selection produced such a high degree of statistical heterogeneity that it was impossible to give a sensible answer. On the other hand, the author's attempt to reduce inconsistency by focusing on a particular intervention in a specific clinical area made a meta-analysis untenable as insufficient studies remained to be accumulated. It is for this reason that there are very few systematic reviews of pain management.

The multidimensional nature of cancer pain

There is now a high level of agreement that the experience of pain consists of three components: the sensory-discriminative, the motivational-affective, and the cognitive-evaluative; with good evidence for the localisation of distinct central pain pathways (Treede *et al.* 1999). There is also consensus that the understanding, assessment, and treatment of an individual's experience of pain requires a biological, social, and psychological perspective (McGuire 1995; Ahles & Martin 1998; Gatchel & Turk 1999). Given the multidimensional nature of cancer pain and the many factors that contribute to individual experience, it is inevitable that a pain management approach that works for one person in a particular setting will not necessarily benefit another, and may not continue to benefit a patient should the environment change. Although not all of the opportunities for inconsistent outcome can be controlled, good practice based on a holistic, multidimensional, interdisciplinary approach takes as many as possible into account. The commonest intervention is that of psychoeducational care – a programme of educational, psychological, and social strategies which has as its aim both treatment and support (Ferrell *et al.* 1993). A typical programme may include:

- instructions about cancer, treatment and living with cancer;
- general information about pain, its assessment and pharmacological treatment aimed at improving adherence to treatment through ensuring that the patient understands the regime, enabling the patient to recognise and manage side-effects, and correcting misconceptions about addiction and tolerance;
- counselling and psychotherapy;
- behavioural approaches to symptom management such as relaxation, imagery, hypnotherapy, cognitive restructuring and problem-solving skills.

Devine & Westlake (1995) systematically reviewed the effectiveness of psychoeducational programmes through a meta-analysis of 116 studies, predominantly from the USA and Canada. Their aim was to evaluate the effects of psychoeducational strategies on psychological and physical well-being, and cancer-related knowledge. The outcomes for psychological well-being were measures of depression and anxiety, and physical well-being was determined by measures of pain and nausea.

Only 13 of the studies reported pain as an outcome and 12 of them showed a positive result. The effect size (ES) based on 11 studies was 0.43, which Cohen (1988) defines as slightly less than 'moderate'. In real terms, this means that the average patient (the one at the statistical mean), after a psychoeducational programme, is reporting less pain than 67 per cent of the control group. This is a modest result. But since the ES has been pooled from a heterogenous sample with a large confidence interval (CI=0.16–0.69), there can be no doubt that some programmes perform better than others. Although the authors did not report effect sizes for individual studies, they did attempt to reduce inconsistency and gain a clearer understanding by examining ES by programme content. The task was handicapped by lack of information in the primary studies about the components that made up the psychoeducational programmes. Two studies were purely educational, and while education greatly enhanced knowledge, it had little effect on pain. Five studies reported the use of relaxation techniques, either alone or in conjunction with music or guided imagery. The aggregated ES was large (d=0.91, CI=0.35–1.47), and homogenous, with the average treated patient reporting less pain than 83 per cent of the untreated group. On the other hand, the four programmes that reported the inclusion of various behavioural strategies were shown to be consistently ineffective.

The potential for diversity in the format and presentation of psychoeducational programmes will inevitably produce clinical heterogeneity. Contributory factors include the number and length of the sessions, the degree of compliance with home practice instructions, and the use and quality of printed material and audiovisual aids. There was insufficient information in the primary studies to examine these effects. Further inconsistency was introduced by inadequate assessment and inclusion criteria. Although one might reasonably assume that patients in the primary studies actually had a pain problem, it cannot be taken for granted. Since pre-treatment levels of pain were not reported, the appropriateness of pain as a measure of outcome cannot be judged. The effect of pre-treatment status is quite clear when one considers the outcomes for nausea. Twenty-six out of 27 studies reported a positive result with an effect size of 0.69. Once again, this was a heterogeneous finding. Restricting the analysis to patients who actually reported nausea prior to the intervention yielded a large and homogenous effect (d=1.04, CI=0.69–1.39).

The problem of relaxation

If relaxation is consistently a component of effective psychoeducational programmes, its effectiveness when used alone remains unproven. Kate Seers and Dawn Carroll recently published two systematic reviews of relaxation; one for acute (Seers & Carroll 1998) and the other for chronic pain (Carroll & Seers 1998). They excluded from their reviews studies in which relaxation was used in combination with cognitive behavioural therapy, biofeedback, hypnosis, or imagery.

In acute pain they identified just seven RCTs that had more than ten subjects, used relaxation as the sole intervention, and reported pain as an outcome. One hundred and fifty patients received relaxation of one type or another. Because of lack of primary data, a meta-analysis was not possible and effect sizes were not calculated. Only two out of the seven studies reported a statistically significant improvement in sensory pain; and three reported significant outcomes for the emotional component of pain.

The authors generously concluded that there was only weak evidence to support the use of relaxation for acute pain.

In chronic pain Carroll & Sears (1998) found nine RCTs that satisfied their inclusion criteria, involving 414 patients, 196 of whom received relaxation. Two of the studies were from oncology (Graffam & Johnson 1987; Sloman *et al.* 1994). Only three of the nine studies, including one of the two cancer studies (Sloman *et al.* 1994), demonstrated relaxation to be superior to experimental control. Although the other oncology study found a significant treatment effect for taped sessions of relaxation, it was no better than the control condition of taped guided imagery. It is of particular note that Sloman *et al.* also provided one group of patients with audiotapes, which again proved to have a positive effect, but relaxation sessions taught by nurses were significantly superior.

Reporting on these systematic reviews *Bandolier*, the much loved tabloid, declared, 'Relax? – don't do it' (Anon 1998). What it should have said was, 'Relax? – do it to music'. Good (1996) undertook a systematic review of the effect of music and relaxation on post-operative pain. She included eleven RCTs, eight non-RCTs, and two further trials without control groups. Fifty per cent of the studies (6/12) that reported a measure for sensory pain found a positive outcome. A significant outcome for affective pain was reported in 77 per cent of studies (10/13). Since non-RCTs can inflate effects by up to 41 per cent (Schultz *et al.* 1995), it is important to consider the results of RCTs separately. The difference is slight: 44 per cent of the RCTs (4/9) reported a significant reduction in sensory pain, and 80 per cent (8/10) for affective pain. Good concludes that relaxation is generally effective for affective pain but equivocal for sensory pain.

The authors of these three reviews note that there are many inconsistencies both within and between studies. The mode of delivery varies from individual or group sessions, to merely presenting the patient with a relaxation tape. The length and the number of sessions were not always reported, and neither was the level of relaxation achieved by the patient, nor the training and ability of the staff. There is also a wide variety of interventions that pass for relaxation, ranging from autogenic training, progressive muscle relaxation, to watching fish. Although many researchers take an atheoretical, pragmatic approach, there are also a number of theoretical rationales. Each relies upon a different mechanism and intervening variable, such as the reduction of muscular tension, the reduction of autonomic arousal and distraction (see Turk *et al.* 1983). Since relaxation cannot be considered to be a unitary phenomenon, it is essential that authors of primary studies specify the technique and the rationale as well as reporting changes in the intervening variable.

Cognitive coping strategies

Fernandez & Turk (1989) define cognitive coping strategies as techniques that covertly influence pain through the medium of thoughts. These include attentional processes, images and statements that patients make about themselves and their experience of pain. Wack & Turk (1984) have identified over 250 cognitive coping strategies, including relaxation, that subjects have used spontaneously in laboratory pain induction studies. The problem of clinical heterogeneity is helped if this large number of strategies can be reduced to a smaller number of categories. Using techniques for multidimensional scaling and cluster analysis, Wack & Turk (1984) identified eight categories of cognitive coping: pleasant imaginings, rhythmic cognitive activity, external focus of attention, pain acknowledging, dramatised coping, neutral imaginings, breathing activity and behavioural activity.

Fernandez & Turk (1989) used the first six categories, so excluding relaxation, to search for primary studies published between 1960 and August 1988 for meta-analysis. Dramatised coping was later dropped from the analysis, as the literature search yielded only a single study. Studies that did not focus on the sensory experience of pain, and those where cognitive strategies were used in combination with some other strategy or intervention were excluded. Only 45 laboratory and two clinical studies were eventually included in a meta-analysis. Overall 85 per cent of the studies reported a positive outcome with an aggregated ES of 0.51 (95% CI=0.42–0.60). Although the strength of laboratory studies lies in their ability to increase internal validity, there still remained a large and significant degree of heterogeneity with individual effect sizes ranging from -0.66 to 1.99. Calculating effect sizes for individual categories did not achieve any degree of consistency. Each category yielded a heterogeneous result with no statistically significant differences between them. Undaunted, the authors produced a league table of relative efficacy (see Table 2.1).

Imagery techniques were the most effective, and pain acknowledging the least. This finding was explained by recourse to the theoretical concept of 'limited capacity' models of attention. The model assumes that attentional capacity is finite, and that when there are competing stimuli, attention becomes selective by filtering out part of the incoming information. Cognitive coping strategies may be seen as impinging on the amount of attention available for nociception. That is to say, distraction displaces the processing of nociceptive information and so attenuates the experience of pain (McCaul & Malott 1984). The theory proposes then that imagery has the greatest analgesic effect because it makes the greatest demand on attentional processes, so

Table 2.1 Relative efficacy of cognitive coping strategies

Cognitive coping strategy	Effect size
Neutral imaginings	0.74
Pleasant imaginings	0.64
External focus of attention	0.49
Rhythmic cognitive activity	0.44
Pain acknowledging	0.34

Source: Fernandez & Turk (1989)

producing greater distraction from pain. Pain acknowledging is the least effective because it is not a distraction task. On the contrary, it requires one to attend to the sensation of pain.

This theoretical explanation was applied *post hoc* and it is by no means certain that it is either true or valid. Eysenck (1995) comments that 'concern with the truth or falsity of a given theory should make us look not at some measurement of effect size but rather at apparent anomalies and contradictions in the data, and at possible explanations of such contradictions'.

The contradiction in this review is that the two clinical studies reverse the general finding. The effect of pain acknowledging was large (d=0.79), whereas the effect of external focus of attention was small (d=0.38). Leventhal (1992) suggests that this is not an anomaly but a significant difference. Laboratory-induced pain has an abrupt onset and is of short duration. It is in some ways similar to dental procedures but not at all like cancer pain. Therefore distraction through competing attentional demands may be effective in some situations and not others.

An alternative view is that distraction works by reducing the affective component of pain (Hodes *et al.* 1990). Anxiety increases attending to pain, which in turn reduces tolerance (Arntz *et al.* 1991). The patient who is extremely anxious about pain may be unable to divert attention and suffer with increased anxiety as a result of trying and failing. On the other hand, acknowledging pain may lead to a reduction in anxiety through the re-interpretation of the meaning of the pain. Furthermore, the individual motivated by fear will avoid anticipated pain and painful activities leading to the desynchronisation of the experience of pain, autonomic response, and behaviour. This can then result in exaggerated pain perception (Rachman & Hodgson 1974). Pain acknowledging may help to restore a more realistic appraisal, and acceptance of pain over time. The key measure then becomes pain tolerance rather than pain threshold. Fernandez & Turk (1989) fail to report which outcome is used in the primary studies.

When there is a high level of heterogeneity in a systematic review there must remain a high level of doubt about the mechanisms that underlie any positive effect. Any theory under test should be clearly stated a priori, and be a criterion for the selection of the studies in the systematic review. The nature of the theory will have considerable impact upon the design of the experimental procedure. For example, if anxiety is not considered to be an important factor, then researchers may not control for it.

The effect of sensory and procedural information on patients

An early study by Egbert *et al.* (1964) found that patients who were told what was going to happen to them and how they could expect to feel after surgery, and were also instructed in what they could do to remain comfortable after the operation, required less medication, and were discharged earlier than patients in the control group. Now that it is obligatory in the UK to obtain a patient's informed consent clinicians are presented with what might be a therapeutic opportunity. On the other hand, there is the view that it is better not to alarm the patient: tell the truth but say as little as possible, and certainly do not raise the expectation of post-operative pain (Langer *et al.* 1975).

Suls & Wan (1989) undertook a systematic review to determine the effect of sensory and procedural information on coping with stressful procedures and pain. They found 21 studies that compared sensory information with no-instruction controls, procedural information with no-instruction controls, and the effect of combining sensory and procedural information. Five of the studies were laboratory-based. They found that there was no difference in the report of self-rated pain between subjects who were given procedural information alone and those who were given no information at all (ES=0.25, CI=-0.15–0.65). Sensory preparation was found to be more effective than control but only modestly so (ES=0.38, CI=0.01–0.075). The combination of sensory and procedural information was found to produce a large and homogenous effect (ES=1.03, CI=0.40–1.65). Suls & Wan suggest that, in combination, sensory information assures that the procedural information is not construed in threatening terms. The procedural information acts in turn as a framework by providing specific events upon which the sensory information can be mapped.

Conclusions and recommendations

As the Editor of the *BMJ* puts it, the primary role of systematic reviews is 'to clear up the Augean stables of medical information' (Smith 1997). The task is about 99 per cent complete once primary studies have been assessed for quality. A good-quality trial is one that removes the likelihood of bias. McQuay & Moore (1998) have developed a simple five-point scale to assess the likelihood of bias in pain research reports. They find that just three items – randomisation, drop-outs and double-blinding – are sufficient to weight the quality of a trial. A study is only appropriately randomised if patients have an equal chance to be included in the trial and if the investigators are unable to predict the next patient to be included. Therefore, picking every other patient or using hospital numbers is inadequate and the study should be excluded from a systematic review. The number and the reason for drop-out should be stated. They also insist on double-blinding, which is impractical for most pain management procedures.

Publication is another significant source of bias. Stern & Simes (1997) found that studies with a positive outcome had a greater chance of being published, and sooner, than studies that report a negative finding. Simes (1986) has made a strong case for an international registry of clinical trials. This is now being actively pursued by the Cochrane Collaboration and the *BMJ*. Meanwhile, a prospective register of controlled trials is published on the internet by Current Science at www.controlled-trials.com. Prospective registration at an early stage can also help reduce clinical heterogeneity by providing a framework for collaboration between systematic reviewers and those undertaking trials in the health service.

Bibliography

Chalmers I & Altman DG (ed.) (1995). *Systematic reviews*. BMJ Publishing Group, London.

McQuay H & Moore A (1998). *An evidence-based resource for pain relief*. Oxford University Press, Oxford.

References

Ahles TA & Martin JB (1992). Cancer pain: a multidimensional perspective. *Hospice Journal* **8**, 25–48.

Anon (1998). Relax? – don't do it. *Bandolier* **53**.

Arntz A, Dressen L & Merckelbach H (1991). Attention not anxiety influences pain. *Behaviour Research & Therapy* **29**, 41–50.

Carroll D & Seers K (1998). Relaxation techniques for chronic pain management: a systematic review. *Journal of Advanced Nursing* **27**, 487.

Cohen J (1988). *Statistical power analysis for the behavioral sciences* 2nd edn. Academic Press, New York, USA.

Devine EC & Westlake SK (1995). The effects of psychoeducational care provided to adults with cancer: meta-analysis of 116 studies. *Oncology Nursing Forum* **22**, 1369–81.

Egbert LD, Batit G, Welch CE & Bartlett MK (1964). Reduction of postoperative pain by encouragement and instruction of patients: a study of doctor-patient rapport. *New England Journal of Medicine* **270**, 825–7.

Eysenck HJ (1995). Problems with meta-analysis. In *Systematic reviews* (ed. I Chalmers & DG Altman), pp. 64–74. BMJ Publishing Group, London.

Fernandez E & Turk DC (1989). The utility of cognitive coping strategies for altering pain perception: a meta-analysis. *Pain* **38**, 123–35.

Ferrell BR, Rhiner M & Ferrell BA (1993). Development and implementation of a pain education program. *Cancer* **72**, 3426–32.

Gatchel RJ & Turk DC (1999). *Psychosocial factors in pain: critical perspectives*. Guilford Press, New York, USA.

Good M (1996). Effect of relaxation and music on postoperative pain: a review. *Journal of Advanced Nursing* **24**, 905–14.

Graffam S & Johnson A (1987). A comparison of two relaxation strategies for relief of pain and its distress. *Journal of Pain and Symptom Management* **2**, 229–31.

Greenhalgh T (1997). How to read a paper: papers that summarise other papers (systematic reviews and meta-analyses). *BMJ* **315**, 672–5.

Hodes RL, Howland EW, Lightfoot N & Cleeland CS (1990). The effects of distraction on responses to cold pressor pain. *Pain* **41**, 109–14.

Langer EJ, Janis IL & Wolfer JA (1975). Reduction of psychological stress in surgical patients. *Journal of Experimental Social Psychology* **11**, 155–65.

Leventhal H (1992). I know distraction works even though it doesn't. *Health Psychology* **11**, 208–9.

McCaul KD & Malott JM (1984). Distraction and coping with pain. *Psychological Bulletin* **95**, 516 33.

McGuire DB (1995). The multiple dimensions of cancer pain: a framework for assessment and management. In *Cancer pain management* (ed. DB McGuire, CH Yarbro & BR Ferrell), pp.1–17. Jones and Bartlett Publishers, Boston, USA.

McQuay H & Moore A (1998). *An evidence-based resource for pain relief*. Oxford University Press, Oxford.

NIH Technology Assessment Panel. (1996). Integration of behavioral and relaxation approaches into the treatment of chronic pain and insomnia. *Journal of the American Medical Association* **276**, 313–18.

Rachman S & Hodgson R (1974). Synchrony and desynchrony in fear and avoidance. *Behaviour Research and Therapy* **12**, 311–18.

Sackett D, Richardson WS, Rosenberg W & Haynes B (1996). *Evidence-based medicine.* Churchill Livingstone, London.

Schultz KF, Chalmers I, Hayes RJ, & Altman DG (1995). Empirical evidence of bias. Dimensions of methodological quality associated with estimates of treatment effects in controlled trials. *Journal of the American Medical Association* **273**, 408–12.

Seers K & Carroll D (1998). Relaxation techniques for acute pain management: a systematic review. *Journal of Advanced Nursing* **27**, 466–75.

Simes RJ (1986). Publication bias: the case for an international registry of clinical trials. *Journal of Clinical Oncology* **4**, 1529–41.

Sindhu F (1996). Are non-pharmacological nursing interventions for the management of pain effective? A meta-analysis. *Journal of Advanced Nursing* **24**, 1152–9.

Sloman R, Brown P, Aldana E & Chee E (1994). The use of relaxation for the promotion of comfort and pain relief in persons with advanced cancer. *Contemporary Nurse* **3**, 6–12.

Smith R (1997). Editor's choice: doctors' information: excessive, crummy, and bent [Editorial]. *BMJ* **315** (7109).

Stern JM & Simes RJ (1997). Publication bias: evidence of delayed publication in a cohort study of clinical research projects. *BMJ* **315**, 640–5.

Suls J & Wan CK (1989). Effects of sensory and procedural information on coping with stressful medical procedures and pain: a meta-analysis. *Journal of Consulting & Clinical Psychology* **57**, 372–9.

Treede R-D, Kenshalo DR, Gracely RH & Jones AKP (1999). The cortical representation of pain. *Pain* **79**, 105–11.

Turk DC, Meichenbaum D & Genest M (1983). *Pain and behavioural medicine: a cognitive-behavioural perspective.* Guilford Press, New York, USA.

Wack JT & Turk DC (1984). Latent structures in strategies for coping with pain. *Health Psychology* **3**, 27–43.

Chapter 3

Decision making at the bedside.
What constitutes 'best medical practice' in the management of cancer pain?

Richard Hillier and Bee Wee

Introduction

Reading Sackett *et al.*'s *Clinical Epidemiology: A basic science for clinical medicine* when it was first published in 1985 was inspiring – not only for 'doers' of research, but especially for 'users' of research. A particular attraction was the book's dedication to, among others, HL Mencken, the great American humorist. A further intriguing dedication was to 'the Emperor's new clothes'. Next, an attractively humorous preface, written by obvious enthusiasts, led the reader on. Like many others, we finished the book with a new commitment to 'the science of the art of medicine' – a more systematic way of gathering and interpreting clinical evidence. In short, though I did not know it then, with a commitment to rigour.

Of course, one has used evidence for many years and has worked with researchers and clinicians who had impressive analytical and research minds. However, for most practitioners in busy clinical posts, finding reliable evidence was time-consuming, while the evidence available was often incomplete and inadequate. Sackett *et al.* had now described in a readable and entertaining manner a systematic but exciting approach which was both pragmatic and attractive to clinicians. More than that, they made it respectable not to do things that did not work, not to do things which others thought might work and, above all, not to do new things without evidence that they did work. Trying the latest new drug or intervention, merely to be seen to be 'with it', was not acceptable. We did not need to wear 'the Emperor's new clothes'.

Subsequently, Sackett *et al.* and their colleagues abroad, notably in Canada, began to systematise evidence by searching the literature to identify all the clinically relevant research, from both basic sciences and clinical research, to bring a more precise analysis to clinical examination, investigation and prognosis. They also examined the effects – both good and bad – of therapeutic intervention. By questioning long-held beliefs, these researchers supported or, more often, refuted them. This was a major advance.

But there was another side to evidence, which, though mentioned, did not have great force in these texts. This was evidence that was based on the clinical experience of what we might call 'good doctors': those colleagues whose knowledge, judgement and even wisdom are valued. If it is true that 'the art of medicine, of being a good doctor or a good nurse – probably, the art of being good at anything – is judgement' (SCOPME 1999), then might this not also be true in the evaluation of evidence?

Unfortunately, unlike good clinical research, it is difficult to define precisely what the characteristics of these 'good doctors' are. There is a danger that they are senior colleagues whom we trust in one field but perhaps should not trust in another, or they may be clinicians who make and carry through judgements by weight of their personalities. This is where the rigour of judgement (art of medicine) meets the rigour of objective measurement (science of medicine). Implicit in this is the crucial assumption that while we must avoid the tyranny of bad science, we must also avoid the dangers of unfounded belief. Good clinicians combine the art and science of medicine all the time. The hallmark of the best professional is the ability to work in the 'messy' reality, where objective facts have to be interpreted using sound professional judgement. The objective facts alone are inadequate for capturing the uniqueness of each clinical encounter. The best clinical practice cannot be achieved by 'science' or 'art' alone. They must be used synergistically and together.

A healthy scepticism should protect us from wishful thinking. It should be remembered that: 'Some drugs work in some situations; sometimes some drugs just don't work'. Oliver Wendell Holmes (1968) was even more sceptical when he suggested that 'if the whole materia medica as used now could be sunk to the bottom of the sea, it would be better for mankind – if worse for the fishes'.

At a more recent conference (reported in a personal communication), when evidence-based medicine was beginning to attract enthusiastic support, Kerr White maintained that 'only about 15–20 per cent of physicians' interventions were supported by the objective evidence that these interventions did more good than harm'. Archie Cochrane, who was also present, is alleged to have called out, 'Kerr, you're a damned liar, you know it isn't more than 10 per cent'. This questioned how much is, or is not, supported by objective evidence. If only 20 per cent of interventions are evidence-based, it follows that 80 per cent of interventions are either of no use or unproven or possibly harmful. Quite a challenge for doctors. None of us wants to think that we might be wasting 80 per cent of our working day.

While the Cochrane Centre emphasises the crucial importance of the randomised controlled trial (RCT) as the basis for evidence, it also concedes the part played by clinical experience and judgement. Unfortunately, exponents of the RCT sometimes overlook or even ridicule the part played by experience which, not surprisingly, has caused considerable antipathy. This is especially true of those areas where precise outcomes are not available, palliative care being an excellent example.

The antipathy in some quarters to evidence-based medicine may have encouraged Ellis *et al.* (1995) to suggest that although only 53 per cent of primary treatments were supported by RCTs, a further 29 per cent had team 'unanimity' in what they described as 'convincing non-experimental evidence'. They maintained that this too should inform the evidence base. Convincing non-experimental evidence included interventions which were 'obvious'. For example, a patient in pain requires pain killers and a patient in urinary retention should be catheterised.

So how, given these dilemmas, do we move forward in basing our clinical practice on reliable and sustainable information?

From ignorance to 'certainty'

In 1983, Hugh Dudley proposed a model of how one might progress from a state of ignorance to a state of relative certainty. Figure 3.1 is adapted from Dudley's (1983) proposals. They run as follows. A chance observation leads the rigorous observer to organise the observations in a systematic way. This, in turn, leads to more complex investigation, systematic reviews through to relative certainty. The key message is that the journey from one to another is a gradual, collaborative, and often quite slow, process in which each stage is valued for its own sake but does not claim to be more than it really is. Each step contributes to the whole and the experienced clinician who is a good observer is often the prime initiator; while the academic scientific team has the infrastructure necessary for the more complex trials and investigations. This is not either/or. Both approaches are needed, if the patient is to benefit. To recognise this turns negative tension between the two groups into an exciting, stimulating and collaborative approach. The only absolute criterion is that each, in its own way, is both rigorous and honest.

So what is it that informs professionals in making decisions at the bedside? Fish & Coles (1998) described a model of what constitutes professional judgement as opposed to technical expertise. They used the concept of professionalism as an iceberg (Figure 3.2). The tip of the iceberg, visible above water level, represents only one-seventh of the mass of the total iceberg. In professional practice, the tip

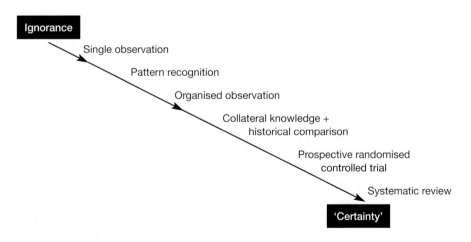

Source: Dudley (1983)

Figure 3.1 From ignorance to 'certainty'

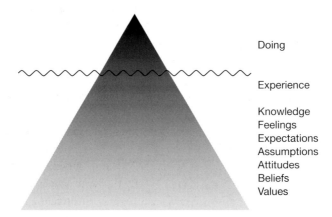

Doing

Experience

Knowledge
Feelings
Expectations
Assumptions
Attitudes
Beliefs
Values

Source: Fish & Coles (1998)

Figure 3.2 Iceberg concept

represents what is seen, ie. the 'act', not the thinking and judgement that underpin it. The tip is therefore what the professional is seen to do.

The portion of the iceberg beneath the water level represents all the elements which, although not visible, are crucial in the making of any professional judgement. It is these that help us function effectively in the messy reality of clinical practice. The professional who has fully developed the qualities which are below the surface, and so are not visible, often gives the impression that what they do is simple. However, if this complexity is not appreciated, only the technical 'recipe' of what they do may be passed on to others who have yet to develop the essential qualities that underpin the best professional practice. If that happens, the iceberg is in danger of overturning, i.e. the balance is wrong and the professional practice is not sustainable.

At the bedside

Keeping the iceberg concept in mind, we can now tease out the process of decision making that occurs at the bedside and the professionalism which enables our technical knowledge to be at its most effective. For example, the technical aspect of prescribing morphine is straightforward; any doctor can write a 'correct' prescription. However, the process of negotiating this with the patient, agreeing the appropriate dosage, allaying anxieties and communicating with the team requires much more than simple pharmacological knowledge.

First, it requires the clinician to create the 'right environment', which includes establishing a rapport with the patient and assessing the 'mood' of the situation. In evaluating the problem, the clinician relies not only on good communication skills, but also on their experience and perceptiveness. The clinician needs to be able to hear what is *not* being said and to have the know-how to check this out sensitively with the patient. All this leads to the working plan which, in the case of diagnosis, can then be confirmed with targeted examination and investigation.

The next step is, arguably, the most testing step for the professional, who now has to make a series of clinical judgements – what to do, when to do it and whether or not to rely on one's own clinical intuition, rather than wait for tests. This is when the professional really needs to draw on those 'invisibles' – the bits of the iceberg underneath the water level. Both clinical effectiveness and the best possible outcome for that particular patient depend on the quality of that judgement.

Clinicians with less experience may be tempted to offer patients a range of options without adequate guidance. In the current climate of patient empowerment, patients are sometimes in danger of being swamped with so much information and choice that they cannot make an informed decision. The patient knows about the patient. The professional should know about the condition. If, on making a decision, the professional uses the whole 'iceberg' approach, the patient will be able to participate in professional practice at its best.

Fashions in evidence

Recently, Campbell & Johnson (1999) explored the nature of fashion in medical education. The model they described can equally apply to fashion in evidence (Figure 3.3). Over-reliance on hard science and anecdote, undue emphasis on the culture of the particular organisation and uncritical use of the literature to support one's position while ignoring clinical reality, all lead to suboptimal professional practice. The greatest

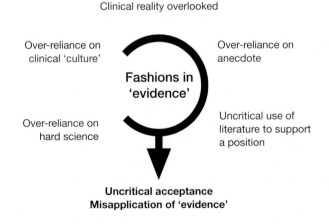

Source: Adapted from Campbell & Johnson (1999)

Figure 3.3 Fashions in evidence

danger of fashion is that not only do clinicians themselves provide suboptimal care, it also encourages others to follow suit. Rigour is lost and with it goes true professionalism. Not only may the patient suffer, but the integrity of the professional is also at risk.

Conclusions

In the current analytical climate of evidence-based medicine and the quest for clinical excellence, both of which will, or should be, supported by clinical governance, we need to answer the question, first formulated by Kenny (1997):

'Is it good science that makes good medicine?' *or*

'Is medicine a human endeavour which employs science?'

It behoves 'good doctors' to value and develop equally the art and the science of medicine in their professional practice and, by developing the 'science of the art of medicine', deliver to the patient the 'art of the science of medicine'. It is this that makes medicine a human endeavour which employs science and, incidentally, what clinical governance should value.

References

Campbell JK & Johnson C (1999). Trend spotting: fashions in medical education. *BMJ* **318**, 1272–5.

Dudley HAF (1983). The controlled clinical trial and the advance of reliable knowledge: an outsider looks in. *British Medical Journal* **287**, 957–60.

Ellis J, Mulligan I, Rowe J & Sackett DL (1995). Inpatient general medicine is evidence based. *Lancet* **346**, 407–10.

Fish D & Coles C (1998). *Developing professional judgement in health care.* Butterworth Heinemann, Oxford.

Holmes OW (1968). In *Familiar medical quotations* (ed. MB Strauss), p.124. Little, Brown, Boston, USA.

Kenny NP (1997). Does good science make good medicine? *Canadian Medical Association Journal* **157**, 33–6.

Sackett DL, Haynes RB & Tugwell P (1985). *Clinical epidemiology: a basic science for clinical medicine.* Little, Brown, Boston, USA.

SCOPME (Standing Committee on Postgraduate Medical and Dental Education) (1999). *Equity and interchange: multiprofessional working and learning.* SCOPME, London.

Chapter 4

Establishing the aetiology of pain. The role of radiological investigation and diagnosis

Allan T Irvine

Introduction

Over the last ten years new imaging modalities and techniques have come into play which allow more rapid and accurate assessment of patients with pain in the palliative care setting. This chapter will deal with the current role of radioisotope imaging, magnetic resonance imaging (MRI), spiral CT and diagnostic ultrasound. Finally, biopsy techniques will be discussed.

A patient with a known malignancy presenting with pain prompts a search for the cause of the pain. Often the pain will be due to local recurrence or metastatic disease. This, in turn, can be broken down into two groups: local recurrence or metastatic disease affecting the skeleton, and those processes affecting soft tissue organs, such as the liver and lymphatic system. This chapter will deal with the current role of radiological investigations in such patients. While local recurrence and metastatic disease should be held uppermost in this setting, it is important to remember that other non-malignant diseases such as cholecystitis, diverticulitis and Paget's disease are all causes of pain that can occur in a known cancer patient. Every effort therefore should be made to establish, first, whether the pain is skeletal or soft tissue in origin and, second, whether it is due to a malignant or a non-malignant process.

Skeletal assessment

For many years nuclear medicine has been a stalwart test for assessment of the skeleton. Non-osseous neoplasms gain access to the skeleton via three mechanisms: by local infiltration; by retrograde venous flow; and via the arterial system. The initial seeding of metastatic disease is in the red marrow, which explains the predominance of metastatic disease in the axial skeleton (Ellis 1961; Russell 1966; Shirazi *et al.* 1974; Tofe 1975; Corcoran *et al.* 1976; Krishnamurthy *et al.* 1977; Rappaport *et al.* 1978; Boyd *et al.* 1984; McNeil 1984; Mobey *et al.* 1984; Tumeh *et al.* 1985; Al Auil *et al.* 1987; Kwai *et al.* 1988; Thrall *et al.* 1987; Boxer *et al.* 1989; Brown 1989; Moore *et al.* 1990).

Radioisotope scanning

As the metastasis grows, the bone remodels through an osteoclastic and osteoblastic reaction. Radioisotope bone scanning needs only a 5–10 per cent change in the lesion-to-bone ratio to be detected on imaging, whereas a 30–50 per cent change is necessary for plain film detection.

In current practice a technetium (Tc) 99m diphosphonate is administered intravenously to the patient. Imaging is undertaken 3–4 hours later. Abnormal patterns for metastatic disease include:

- multiple focal lesions
- solitary lesions
- diffuse involvement (superscan)
- photon-deficient areas
- flare phenomenon.

While sensitive for picking up abnormal areas of activity, the bone scan remains a non-specific investigation. Patients presenting with skeletal pain in the palliative care setting may have alternative processes such as:

- metabolic disease (including osteoporosis, osteomalacia and Cushing's syndrome)
- trauma
- arthritis
- osteomyelitis
- Paget's disease
- bone infarction.

Patients with either solitary lesions or small numbers of lesions present a particular problem in diagnosis (Shirazi 1974; Corcoran *et al.* 1976; Rappaport 1978; Brown 1983). The most common source of confusion is degenerative arthritis, followed next by assessment of a healing fracture.

Another potential pitfall in radioisotope imaging is the superscan. In this condition the whole skeleton has diffuse uptake and the scan may appear deceptively normal. Detection of lesions that cause marrow infiltration without a reactive bone reaction can also occur. This is a particular problem with round cell tumours and multiple myeloma (Kaufman 1978; Thrall *et al.* 1987). The flare phenomenon is an osteoblastic response to treatment, resulting in abnormally increased uptake, which would in the normal course of events be interpreted as progressive disease, when in fact the reverse is true with the disease process responding to treatment (Thomas 1968; Norman *et al.* 1969; Sy *et al.* 1975; Goergen *et al.* 1976; Hemmingsson *et al.* 1979; Sartoris *et al.* 1985; Thrall 1987).

Paget's disease and osteomyelitis are two further conditions which cause confusion in interpretation for metastatic disease. The co-existence of metastatic disease with both these conditions renders radioisotope interpretation difficult.

Direct invasion of the skeleton by the primary tumour or extension from a secondary site such as a lymph node is normally accompanied by a soft tissue mass, which will not be apparent on radioisotope imaging. Haematogeneous spread is much more frequent, and in the spine the venous route, including Batson's paravertebral plexus, appears more important than the arterial one.

There are several mechanisms present which may contribute to the cause of bone pain in metastatic disease. These include the release of chemical mediators, elevated intraosseous pressure, periosteal elevation and incipient or actual pathological fractures. Pain may be a consequence of joint involvement by metastatic disease, which can occur from symptoms due to involvement of adjacent bone, collapse of an articular surface, loss of structural support due to tumour and synovial infiltration (Resnick *et al.* 1988). While these changes may be detected by radioisotope imaging, the appearances will be non-specific.

In addition to malignant invasion, arthritic-type pain may be due to paraneoplastic effects, such as carcinomatous polyarthritis, which simulates rheumatoid symptoms, and other carcinoma-related rheumatic conditions (e.g. Sjogren's syndrome, lupus, dermatomyositis, hypertrophic pulmonary osteoarthropathy, secondary gout and pyogenic arthritis due to streptococcus bovis and clostridium species secondary to bowel cancer) (Resnick 1985). Skeletal changes due to radionecrosis may be difficult to distinguish from metastatic lesions.

As radioisotope accumulates at any skeletal site with an increased bone turnover, it remains a sensitive but non-specific test. This lack of specificity is well recognised and has led to the recommendation that positive scans be accompanied by plain film correlation. As a radioisotope scan is more sensitive than the radiograph, a positive plain film confirms the diagnosis of tumour, whereas a negative plain film does not exclude it.

SPECT

In recent years there have been advances in radioisotope techniques that have improved metastatic detection. These advances include single photon emission computed tomography (SPECT), which can improve sensitivity and specificity of radioisotope bone imaging (Ryan *et al.* 1995), and positron emission tomography (PET), using fluorodeoxyglucose (FDG), which detects abnormal areas of glucose metabolism, although its role in clinical practice is not yet established (Ryan *et al.* 1995; Dehdashti 1996; Shreve *et al.* 1996).

Bone marrow may be labelled with Tc 99m colloid to evaluate the state of haematopoiesis and phagocytic activity; however, it has proved to be a non-specific test and does not clearly distinguish between normal and abnormal marrow (Datz *et al.* 1985; Vogler *et al.* 1988; Widding *et al.* 1989; Steiner *et al.* 1990; Algra *et al.* 1992).

Bone marrow scanning has been reported to be more sensitive than conventional radioisotope bone imaging in metastatic prostate cancer (Reske 1991) and in urological malignancy using Tc 99m anti-NCA-95 monoclonal antibody. For certain primary soft tissue tumours such as lymphomas and sarcomas scanning with gallium may be a useful tool (Finn *et al.* 1987; Southee *et al.* 1992).

Computed tomography

CT scanning has had a limited impact on the detection of skeletal metastases. While it is more sensitive than plain film for the detection of tumour, it is not a practical tool for assessing the whole skeleton. In view of its suboptimal discrimination between normal and abnormal bone marrow, along with streak and beam hardening artefacts from cortical bone, its role is chiefly in confirming suspicious areas identified with radioisotope imaging and for biopsy planning (Helms *et al.* 1981; Steiner *et al.* 1993).

MRI

Magnetic resonance imaging (MRI) is highly sensitive to skeletal metastases, in part because of its ability to demonstrate abnormalities in bone marrow. This is because of its ability to separate fat from other tissues. Because of its advantages, MRI has assumed a critical role in the detection of metastatic disease (Daffner *et al.* 1986; Moore *et al.* 1986; Widding *et al.* 1987; Linden *et al.* 1988; Negendank *et al.* 1990).

Cancellous or spongy bone is composed of primary and secondary trabeculae, which act as a framework for bone marrow. Blood supply is via the nutrient and periosteal arterial systems with venous drainage through a sinusoidal network. The adolescent marrow is composed of 40 per cent water, 40 per cent fat and 20 per cent protein. With increasing age, the fat level increases so that a 70-year-old will have cellular marrow consisting of 30 per cent water, 60 per cent fat and 10 per cent protein. This fatty marrow has a relatively sparse blood supply. This process of change from a rich vascular marrow (red marrow) to a fatty marrow is termed 'marrow conversion'. Although metastatic disease occurs throughout the marrow, it is more frequently encountered in the cellular marrow because of its rich vascularity.

MRI is sensitive to tumour infiltration, particularly on T1 and STIR images, because of the high contrast resolution between water and fat. Lytic metastases are characterised by low signal on T1-weighted images and high signal on STIR images. Sclerotic deposits with an osteoblastic appearance will give rise to low signal on all pulse sequences (Trillet *et al.* 1989; Algra *et al.* 1992). Metastatic deposits are usually well defined and are frequently associated with a small zone of oedema, a distinguishing feature from osteomyelitis or a fracture in which significant oedema is present.

Like radioisotopes, MRI remains a relatively insensitive investigation, however. In one study (Hanna *et al.* 1991), MRI scans were compared with histological specimens at 21 sites, 7 of which contained tumour and 14 of which did not. For all the positive tumour sites, abnormalities were revealed on the MRI scans. However, of the sites shown to be free of tumour, there was a significant (more than 50 per cent in some instances) false positive rate due to the inability of MRI to distinguish tumour from the effects of treatment. However, MRI can demonstrate metastases that are not apparent on radioisotope bone scans (Kattapuram *et al.* 1990; Colletti *et al.* 1991). It is particularly well suited to detecting spinal metastases. Because MRI can detect soft tissue changes, any spinal compression can be readily assessed, and it has become the standard investigation for suspected cord compression.

Conclusion

Radioisotopes offer a large field of view, inexpensive radiopharmaceuticals and low morbidity. MRI is a simple and faster method for evaluating the axial skeleton but is less suited to screening the long bones. There are, however, significant contraindications to MRI – notably, patients with pacemakers and certain ferromagnetic vascular clips, or those who suffer from claustrophobia.

Soft tissue assessment

In establishing the aetiology of pain arising from soft tissue structures the key investigations are ultrasound and X-ray CT. Both are cross-sectional imaging techniques, which give comparable results.

Diagnostic ultrasound gives a rapid, non-invasive assessment of the head and neck, abdomen and pelvis. Its major limitations are that it is operator-dependent and that assessment of deep-lying structures in the abdomen, such as the retroperitoneum, and the presence of bowel gas reduce its effectiveness.

Soft tissue assessment ultrasound

Head and neck ultrasound

With the advent of higher frequency probes (7.5–15 MHz) more accurate assessment of soft tissue structures of the neck has become possible. The size, texture and changes in the thyroid gland and salivary glands with the assessment of lymphadenopathy are well established. However, the newer probes can now identify small structures, such as the vagus and recurrent laryngeal nerves. The main signs for local malignant invasion with ultrasound are strap muscle infiltration and encasement of vascular and nerve structures.

Normal lymph nodes are not usually identified on ultrasound as their echogenicity is similar to that of subcutaneous fat. Reactive or neoplastic nodes are usually larger and less echogenic, rendering them visible to ultrasound assessment.

Any lymph node of over 5 mm in an axial diameter is considered abnormal in the neck. The differentiation between reactive and neoplastic nodes is difficult. The former tend to maintain an oval shape, whereas the latter become more rounded. The 'roundness index' (RI) is obtained by dividing the longitudinal by the axial diameter and may be of some use. In one study 71 per cent of nodes with an RI smaller than 1.5 were malignant, whereas 84 per cent of nodes with a ratio of greater than 2 were reactive. (Sakai 1988; Hajek *et al.* 1990; Solbiati *et al.* 1992).

Abdomen and pelvis

The liver, spleen, pancreas and para-aortic region are readily assessed by ultrasound examination. Ultrasound is a well-established technique for the assessment of primary or metastatic disease for major organs. In the context of pain, subcapsular infiltration or involvement of coeliac axis lymph nodes is relevant and should be noted.

The major advance in ultrasound is the introduction of transvaginal ultrasound in the assessment of the female pelvis. Because of the closer proximity to the uterus and ovaries this technique more closely simulates a bimanual examination, as the examiner's free hand can be used to palpate or move the pelvic organs closer to the field of view. The higher frequencies employed (5–10 MHz) provide improved resolution.

However, large adnexal and other pelvic masses may not be adequately seen because they are either larger than, or outside, the field of view. For this reason conventional or transabdominal scanning is often recommended as a preliminary study prior to transvaginal scanning (TVS).

TVS provides additional information in 16–60 per cent of patients over transabdominal scanning. Image quality is improved in 22–87 per cent of scans (Coleman *et al.* 1988; Mendelson *et al.* 1988; Freimanis *et al.* 1992). The patient is examined with an empty bladder. Detailed examination of the uterus, including the endometrium, the adnexal regions and the ovaries is possible. Colour duplex ultrasound can be combined with TVS to assess pelvic masses. As a general rule, malignant masses have a low pulsatility index or a low resistive index. In post-menopausal ovaries, for example, a resistive index of less than 0.5 should arouse suspicion for malignancy (Fleischer 1991).

In a patient with cancer pain the detection of fluid or a mass in the pelvis on TVS may be an indicator of neoplasia or infection. Aspiration, biopsy and transcatheter drainage can be performed under TVS guidance. A needle or catheter assembly can be inserted either transabdominally or via the TV needle guide through the vaginal wall. Using an aseptic technique this is successful in over 90 per cent of cases. In over 86 per cent of patients in one study surgery was avoided using this technique (van Sonnenberg 1991).

Drawbacks of the TV approach include interposed bowel, tough vaginal wall and the difficulty of fixing a catheter in place.

X-ray CT

X-ray CT is a well-established technique for whole body assessment, particularly the head and neck, chest, abdomen and pelvis. It has become a key imaging modality in the cancer patient, both for tumour staging, treatment evaluation and assessment of complications. In a cancer patient with pain it can rapidly give evaluation of soft tissue and bony structures. Unlike ultrasound, it is not operator-dependent and overlying bowel gas and obesity are not obstacles to good imaging. In fact imaging quality is usually improved in the retroperitoneum by the presence of fat. It does involve ionising radiation.

The introduction of volumetric (helical or spiral) scanning has further improved image quality and resolution. Initially reported by Kalender *et al.* (1990), volumetric scanning involves continuous data acquisition while the patient is advanced through the CT gantry. Scans may be either prospectively or retrospectively reconstructed at operator-selected levels. The result is a continuous set of images obtained without interscan delay obviating potential misregistration.

In addition to the usual scanning parameters, spiral CT requires prescribing both the speed of table incrementation and the time of scan duration. Typically, this is within the range of a single respiratory inspiration.

The pitch is defined as the ratio between slice thickness and the rate of table incrementation. Increasing the pitch allows a greater volume to be scanned per unit time. Thus a slice thickness or collimation of 10 mm and a table movement of 10 mm per second gives a pitch of 1.0. An increase of table movement to 20 mm per second while maintaining the slice thickness at 10 mm would give a pitch of 2.0. This would allow a greater overall distance to be travelled in a single breath hold and decrease radiation dose. Small lesion detection may be compromised by increasing pitch to 2.0 or beyond and for this reason a pitch of 1.0–1.5 is usually performed in the setting of malignant disease. Regardless of pitch, spiral CT always results in contiguous images (Brink *et al.* 1992; Costello *et al.* 1992; Polacin *et al.* 1992; Heiken *et al.* 1993).

In comparison with routine axial CT there are a number of important advantages for spiral CT. These include reduced time of the examination and improved multiplanar and 3-D images. The absence of misregistration allows superb multiplanar reconstructions to be generated in any imaging plane (Naidich *et al.* 1993). A further advantage of spiral CT is the ability to obtain images of an organ in both the arterial and venous phases, unlike conventional CT, which could only obtain images in the later venous stage. As a consequence of this and the elimination of respiration-induced misregistration, spiral CT has the potential to detect more lesions than conventional CT (Jones *et al.* 1992; Urban *et al.* 1993; Baumgarten *et al.* 1994).

Percutaneous biopsy

Percutaneous biopsy has become established as a safe and effective procedure. It has been used for most organs with excellent results and few complications (Gazelle *et al.* 1989; Parker *et al.* 1989; Wittich *et al.* 1992). The key to these procedures is image guidance (whether by fluoroscopy, CT, ultrasound or, recently, MRI), which allows, first, a route to be planned into the site for biopsy and, second, to visualise the biopsy needle entering the lesion confirming that the correct area has been sampled.

Percutaneous biopsy is less invasive than surgery and can be applied to patients who are too ill to undergo surgery or wish to avoid convalescence from a diagnostic laparotomy.

When considering percutaneous biopsy it is pertinent to take into account the general condition of the patient, the site, size and accessibility of the lesion, and the potential risk to vital structures around the area to be biopsied. Often these risk factors are cumulative. Biopsy needles which obtain histological cause are available in 18- and 20-gauge, and these will usually suffice. Thinner-gauge needles are available for fine needle aspiration (FNA) procedures.

In the setting of pain in a cancer patient the risk versus the benefit should be considered. Coagulation defects increase risk of bleeding and, if possible, should be corrected prior to biopsy. In some cases there may not be a safe pathway to the lesion, with vital organs and bowel interposed between the skin and the lesion. Traversing bowel and vital organs is not in itself a contraindication to biopsy but should be avoided if possible. In some circumstances, however, it may be inevitable that these structures are traversed.

There is a spectrum of biopsy complexity, ranging from large masses or fluid collections located superficially with no interposing vital structures to smaller seated lesions overlaid by vital organs.

Complications or percutaneous biopsies are of two types, generic and organ-specific. Generic refers to complications that are common to all biopsies and include bleeding, infection and unintended organ damage (Nosher et al. 1982; Chan et al. 1983; Whelen et al. 1985; Baumgarter 1986). Surgical intervention as a consequence of a biopsy complication is under 2 per cent (Murphy et al. 1988; Teplick et al. 1988; Nolsoe 1990) but the risk increases with larger gauge needles (Gazelle et al. 1992; Littrup et al. 1994; Shepard 1994; Watkinson et al. 1994).

Organ-specific complications are those associated with biopsy of a specific organ. For example, pneumothorax is most commonly associated with lung biopsy, but can occur during vertebral, lung and breast biopsy (Goralnik 1988; van Sonnenberg 1988; Wernecke et al. 1989; Ikezoe 1990; Haramati 1991).

At our institution we perform biopsy procedures as both inpatients and outpatients. All our biopsy techniques can be performed as an outpatient procedure. Admission is unnecessary, provided there are facilities to monitor the patient following the procedure. All patients undergoing biopsy are told that they will be kept under observation for 2–4 hours following the procedure. They should have an able-bodied relative to accompany them home. The homeward journey should be by car, taxi or hospital transport, and not by public transport.

Following informed consent, which includes discussion of the relevant complications such as haemorrhage and pneumothorax, the patient is positioned in the fluoroscopic unit, CT scanner or ultrasound table. Intravenous access is obtained for liver, renal and bone biopsies as a route for intravenous sedation and analgesia, as well as a route for resuscitation should this be required. Routine intravenous sedation is not given for soft-tissue organ biopsies, unless the patient is particularly anxious, but is given for bone biopsies. A combination of midazolam and fentanyl is given in these circumstances. If sedation is given, continual pulse oximetry monitoring is mandatory.

Chest biopsy

Pleural-based lesions are best biopsied using CT or ultrasound guidance, whereas fluoroscopy is used for intrapulmonary lesions. The skin overlying the mass is marked using CT, fluoroscopic or ultrasound guidance. Using an aseptic technique, 10 ml of 2 per cent lignocaine is instilled into the skin, subcutaneous tissue and then deeper, if necessary, to any pain-related structures such as the pleura. A co-axial technique is normally used. A short (6 cm) needle of either 16- or 18-gauge is introduced in the direction of the mass. The tip of the small guide needle is checked in relation to the mass and re-adjusted as necessary. For pleural-based lesions an 18-gauge biopsy cutting needle is used, while for intrapulmonary lesions a 20-gauge biopsy cutting needle is required. At least two passes are made through the guide needle and material obtained for histology or microbiology.

An immediate post-procedure CT scan or chest X-ray for fluoroscopic approaches is obtained to assess for early complications, including pneumothorax and pulmonary haemorrhage. If this does not show any abnormality and the patient remains well, then a repeat chest X-ray is not obtained and the patient is allowed home after two hours, accompanied by a friend or relative. A small pulmonary haemorrhage resulting in haemoptysis following the biopsy, although alarming for both the patient and radiologist, normally settles quickly. A small (less than 20 per cent) pneumothorax which does not progress on a second chest X-ray and is asymptomatic does not require further investigation or admission. In these circumstances the patient is allowed home. If the patient has significant pain, shortness of breath or there is concern over the home setting or social factors, then the patient will be admitted for overnight observation.

The patient is given an information sheet detailing the procedure they have undergone. This includes a telephone number that the patient can ring (including an 'on call' number), and the patient is told to return to hospital if they feel unwell, become short of breath or develop increasing chest pain, which might indicate a developing pneumothorax or other complication. The patient's telephone number is obtained and our X-ray nurses ring the patient the following day to check that they are well. Finally, we arrange for a clinic follow-up appointment, normally at one week or earlier, if indicated, when the patient can discuss the biopsy results with the referring clinician.

A copy of the biopsy report is kept and we obtain the histology or microbiology report in all cases. Not only is this useful for audit purposes but allows us to recall the patient for a repeat biopsy prior to their follow-up appointment if the specimen is technically unsatisfactory. This avoids an unnecessary trip for the patient to the referring clinician in the event of an unhelpful biopsy report (Giron *et al.* 1996).

Abdominal and pelvic biopsy

As with the chest biopsy, a co-axial technique is used for abdominal and pelvis biopsy. For ultrasound biopsy a single needle is used as the co-axial technique is unnecessary.

The overlying skin is marked and using aseptic technique a biopsy obtained. Normally an 18-gauge cutting biopsy is used with two passes taken. Following the biopsy, the patient's vital signs are monitored and if the patient remains stable, they are allowed home after two hours. Liver biopsy patients are kept for a longer period of four hours. Following liver biopsy, patients often develop right-sided or shoulder tip pain. Intravenous fentanyl is given, and provided the pain settles and vital signs remain stable, the patient is allowed home. If we feel it is indicated, we perform a bedside ultrasound examination in our recovery unit. The presence of any free fluid within the abdomen is taken as evidence of an intraperitoneal haemorrhage and the patient is admitted for observation even if their vital signs are stable. With the exception of liver biopsy patients, the patient's clotting status is not routinely checked. Patients on oral anticoagulation need either to stop this prior to biopsy or to be switched to heparin. The follow-up procedure detailed for chest biopsy is followed in all abdominal and pelvic biopsies.

Following the procedure, the most telling sign that there has been no complication is that of the impatient patient, wanting to go home. Even so, we insist that the patient remain under observation for the specified time. Food and liquid refreshment are permitted during the observation period, providing the patient is stable.

Conclusion

Radiological investigations play a key role in the assessment of pain in a cancer patient. Initial investigations should be directed towards whether the pain is skeletal or soft tissue in origin. Once this has been done, then specific tests can be undertaken to elucidate whether the cause of the pain is due to a neoplastic or non-neoplastic cause. In some instances percutaneous biopsy will be necessary for histological diagnosis.

References

Alavi A *et al.* (1987). Scintigraphic examination of bone and marrow infarcts in sickle cell disorders. *Semin Roentgenol* **22**, 213.

Algra PR & Bloem JL (1992). Magnetic resonance imaging of metastatic disease and multiple myeloma. In *MRI and CT of the musculoskeletal system* (ed. JL Bleom & DJ Sartoris), p. 218. Williams and Wilkins, Baltimore, USA.

Baumgarten D *et al.* (1994). *Spiral CT of the liver: comparison of the focal hepatic detection rate using 5x5-mm and 5x10-mm collimation.* American Roentgen Ray Society, New Orleans, USA.

Baumgartner NL & Bernadino ME (1986). Percutaneous renal biopsies: accuracy, safety, and indications. *Urol Radiol* **8**, 67–71.

Boxer DI *et al.* (1989). Bone secondaries in breast cancer: the solitary metastasis. *J Nucl Med* **30**, 1318.

Boyd CM *et al.* (1984). Significance of the solitary lesion on bone scans of adults with primary extraosseous cancer [Abstract]. *Radiology* **153P**, 119.

Brink JA *et al.* (1992). Spiral CT, decreased spatial resolution in vivo due to broadening of section-sensitivity profile. *Radiology* **185**, 469–74.

Brown ML (1983). Significance of the solitary lesion in pediatric bone scanning. *J Nucl Med* **24**, 114–15.

Brown ML (1989). The role of radionuclides in the patient with osteogenic sarcoma. *Semin Roentgenol* **24**, 185.

Chan JC *et al.* (1983). Renal biopsies under ultrasound guidance: 100 consecutive biopsies in children. *J Urol* **129**, 103–7.

Coleman BG *et al.* (1988). Transvaginal and transabdominal sonography: prospective comparison. *Radiology* **168**, 639–43.

Colletti PM *et al.* (1991). Spinal MR imaging in suspected metastases: correlation with skeletal scintigraphy. *Magn Reson Imaging* **9**, 349–55.

Corcoran RJ *et al.* (1976). Solitary abnormalities in bone scans of patients with extraosseous malignancies. *Radiology* **121**, 663–7.

Costello P *et al.* (1992). Spiral CT of the thorax with increased table speed, comparative study [Abstract]. *Radiology* **185**, 131.

Daffner RH *et al.* (1986). MRI in the detection of malignant infiltration of bone marrow. *Am J Roentgenol* **146**, 353.

Datz FI & Taylor A Jr (1985). The clinical use of radionuclide bone marrow imaging. *Semin Nucl Med* **15**, 239.

Dehdashti F *et al.* (1996). Benign versus malignant intraosseous lesions, discrimination by means of PET with 2[F-18]fluoro-2-deoxy-d-glucose. *Radiology* **200**, 243–7.

Ellis RE (1961). The distribution of active bone marrow in the adult. *Phys Med Biol* **5**, 255–8.

Finn HA *et al.* (1987). Scintigraphy with gallium-67 citrate in staging of soft-tissue sarcomas of the extremity. *J Bone Joint Surgery* **69**A, 886–91.

Fleischer AC *et al.* (1991). Assessment of ovarian tumour vascularity with transvaginal colour Doppler sonography. *J Ultrasound Med* **10**, 563–8.

Freimanis MG & Jones AF (1992). Transvaginal ultrasonography. *Radiol Clin North Am* **30**, 955–76.

Gazelle GS & Haaga JR (1989). Guided percutaneous biopsy of intra-abdominal lesions. *Am J Roentgenol* **153**, 929–35.

Gazelle GS *et al.* (1992). Effect of needle gauge, level of antiocoagulation, and target organ on bleeding associated with aspiration biopsy. *Radiology* **183**, 509–13.

Giron J *et al.* (1996). Interventional chest radiology. *Eur Jour Radiology* **23**, 58–78.

Goergen RG *et al.* (1976). 'Cold' bone lesions: a newly recognized phenomenon of bone imaging. *J Nucl Med* **17**, 184.

Goralnik CH *et al.* (1988). CT-guided cutting needle biopsies of selected chest lesions. *Am J Roentgenol* **151**, 903–7.

Hajek PC *et al.* (1990). Lymph nodes of the neck: evaluation with US. *Radiology* **158**, 739.

Hanna SL *et al.* (1991). Magnetic resonance imaging of disseminated bone marrow disease in patients treated for malignancy. *Skeletal Radiol* **20**, 79–84.

Haramati LB & Austin JHM (1991). Complications after CT-guided needle biopsy through aerated versus non-aerated lung. *Radiology* **181**, 778.

Heiken JP *et al.* (1993). Spiral (helical) CT. *Radiology* **189**, 647–56.

Helms CA *et al.* (1981). Detection of bone marrow metastases using quantitative computed tomography. *Radiology* **140**, 745.

Hemmingsson A *et al.* (1979). Image enhancement by digital-analog filtration. III. Experiences with bone metastases. *Acta Radiol (Diagn)* **20**, 841–6.

Ikezoe J *et al.* (1990). Percutaneous biopsy of thoracic lesions: value of sonography for needle guidance. *Am J Roentgenol* **154**, 1181–5.

Jones EC *et al.* (1992). The frequency and significance of small (≤15mm) hepatic lesions detected by CT. *Am J Roentgenol* **158**, 535–9.

Kalender WA *et al.* (1990). Spiral volumetric CT with single-breath-hold technique, continuous transport, and continuous scanner rotation. *Radiology* **176**, 181–3.

Kattapuram SV *et al.* (1990). Negative scintigraphy with positive magnetic resonance imaging in bone metastasis. *Skeletal Radiol* **19**, 113–16.

Kaufman RA *et al.* (1978). False negative bone scans in neuroblastoma metastatic to the ends of long bones. *Am J Roentgenol* **130**, 131.

Krishnamurthy GT (1977). Distribution pattern of metastatic bone disease: a need for total body skeletal image. *JAMA* **237**, 2504–6.

Kwai AH *et al.* (1988). Clinical significance of isolated scintigraphic sternal lesions in patients with breast cancer. *J Nucl Med* **29**, 324.

Linden A *et al.* (1988). Malignant lymphoma: bone marrow imaging versus biopsy. *Radiology* **173**, 335.

Littrup PJ *et al.* (1994). Prostate biopsy decisions and complications. *Semin Intervent Radiol* **11**, 231–6.

McNeil BJ (1984). Value of bone scanning in neoplastic disease. *Semin Nucl Med* **14**, 277–86.

Mendelson EB *et al.* (1988). Gynecologic imaging: comparison of transabdominal and transvaginal sonography. *Radiology* **166**, 321–4.

Moore SG *et al.* (1986). Bone marrow in children with acute lymphocytic leukemia, MR relaxation times. *Radiology* **160**, 237.

Moore SG *et al.* (1990). Primary disorders of bone marrow. In *Magnetic resonance imaging in children* (ed. MD Cohen & MR Edwards), p.765. BC Decker, Philadelphia, USA.

Murphy FB *et al.* (1988). CT or sonography-guided biopsy of the liver in the presence of ascites: frequency of complications. *Am J Roentgenol* **151**, 485–6.

Naidich DP (1993). Volumetric scans change perceptions in thoracic imaging. *Diagnostic Imaging* **15**, 70–4.

Negendank W *et al.* (1991). Evidence for clonal disease by magnetic resonance imaging in patients with hypoplastic marrow disorders. *Blood* **78**, 2872–9.

Nolsoe C *et al.* (1990). Major complications and deaths due to interventional ultrasonography: a review of 8000 cases. *J Clin Ultrasound* **18**, 179–184.

Norman A & Ulin R (1969). A comparative study of periosteal new-bone response in metastatic bone tumours (solitary) and primary bone sarcomas. *Radiology* **92**, 705–8.

Nosher JL *et al.* (1982). Fine needle aspiration of kidney and adrenal gland. *J Urol* **128**, 896–9.

Parker SH *et al.* (1989). Image-directed percutaneous biopsies with a biopsy gun. *Radiology* **171**, 663–9.

Polacin A *et al.* (1992). Evaluation of section sensitivity profiles and image noise in spiral CT. *Radiology* **185**, 29–35.

Rappaport AH *et al.* (1978). Unifocal bone findings by scintigraphy: clinical significance in patients with known primary cancer. *West J Med* **129**, 188–92.

Reske SN (1991). Recent advances in both marrow scanning skeleton. *Eur J Nucl Med* **3**, 203–21.

Resnick D (1985). Skeletal metastatic disease: its articular manifestations. *Orthop Rev* **5**, 98–104.

Resnick D & Niwayama G (1988). *Diagnosis of bone and joint disorders*. WB Saunders, Philadelphia, USA.

Robey EL & Schellhammer PE (1984). Solitary lesion on bone scan in genitourinary malignancy. *J Urol* **132**, 1000–2.

Russell WJ *et al.* (1966). Active bone marrow distribution in the adult. *Br J Radiol* **39**, 735–9.

Ryan PJ & Fogelman I (1995). The bone scan: where are we now? *Semin Nucl Med* **25**, 76–91.

Sakai F *et al.* (1988). Ultrasonic evaluation of cervical metastastic lymphadenopathy. *J Ultrasound Med* **7**, 305.

Sartoris DJ *et al.* (1985). Preliminary report. Dual-energy scanned projection radiography of osseous metastatic disease. *Invest Radiol* **20**, 983–8.

Shepard JAO (1994). Complications of percutaneous needle aspiration biopsy of the chest: prevention and management. *Semin Intervent Radiol* **11**, 181–6.

Shirazi PH *et al.* (1974). Review of solitary 18F bone scans lesions. *Radiology* **112**, 369–72.

Shreve PD *et al.* (1996). Metastatic prostate cancer: initial findings of PET with 2-deoxy-2-[F18]-fluoro-D-glucose. *Radiology* **199**, 751–6.

Solbiati L *et al.* (1988). High resolution sonography of cervical lymph nodes in head and neck cancer: criteria for differentiation of reactive versus malignant nodes. In *Proceedings of the 74th meeting of the Radiologic Society of North America,* p.113. RSNA, Chicago, Illinois, USA.

Solbiati L *et al.* (1992). Ultrasonography of the neck. *Radiol Clin North Am* **30**, 941–54.

Song HY *et al.* (1996). Lacrimal canalicular obstructions: safety and effectiveness of balloon dilatation 1. *JVIR* **7**, 929–34.

Southee AE *et al.* (1992). Gallium imaging in metastatic and recurrent soft tissue sarcoma. *J Nucl Med* **33**,1594–9.

Steiner RM *et al.* (1990). Magnetic resonance imaging of bone marrow: diagnostic value in diffuse hematologic disorders. *Magn Reson Q* **6**, 17–34.

Steiner RM *et al.* (1993). MRI of diffuse bone marrow disease. *Radiol Clin North Am* **31**, 383–409.

Sy WM *et al.* (1975). Significance of absent or faint kidney sign on bone scan. *J Nucl Med* **16**, 454–6.

Teplick SK *et al.* (1988). Percutaneous pancreaticobiliary biopsies in 173 patients using primarily ultrasound or fluoroscopic guidance. *Cardiovasc Intervent Radiol* **11**, 26–8.

Thomas BM (1968). Three unusual carcinoid tumours with particular reference to osteoblastic bone metastases. *Clin Radiol* **19**, 221–5.

Thrall JH & Byrton (1987). Skeletal metastases. *Radiol Clin North Am* **25**, 1155–70.

Tofe AJ *et al.* (1975). Correlation of neoplasms with incidence and localization of skeletal metastases: an analysis of 1355 diphosphonate bone scans. *J Nucl Med* **16**, 986–9.

Trillet V *et al.* (1989). Bone marrow metastases in small cell lung cancer: detection with magnetic resonance imaging and monoclonal antibodies. *Br J Cancer* **60**, 83–8.

Tumeh SS *et al.* (1985). Clinical significance of solitary rib lesions in patients with extra-skeletal malignancy. *J Nucl Med* **26**, 1140–3.

Urban BA *et al.* (1993). Detection of focal hepatic lesions with spiral CT, comparison of 4- and 8-mm interscan spacing. *Am J Roentgenol* **106**, 783–5.

van Sonnenberg E *et al.* (1988). Difficult thoracic lesions: CT-guided biopsy experience in 150 cases. *Radiology* **167**, 457–61.

van Sonnenberg E *et al.* (1991). US-guided transvaginal drainage of pelvic abscesses and fluid collections. *Radiology* **181**, 53–6.

Vogler JB & Murphy WA (1988). Bone marrow imaging. *Radiology* **168**, 679–93.

Ward HP & Block MH (1971). The natural history of agogenic myeloid metaplasia (AMM) and a critical evaluation of its relationship with the myeloproliferative syndrome. *Medicine* **50**, 357–420.

Watkinson AF & Adam A (1994). Complications of abdominal and retroperitonal biopsy. *Semin Intervent Radiol* **11**, 254–66.

Wernecke K *et al.* (1989). Mediastinal tumours: biopsy under US guidance. *Radiology* **172**, 473–6.

Whelen TV *et al.* (1985). Renal biopsy: localization using computed tomography. *Urol Radiol* **7**, 94–6.

Widding A *et al.* (1989). Bone marrow investigative with technetium-99m microcolloid and magnetic resonance imaging in patients with malignant myelolympho-proliferative disease. *Eur J Nucl Med* **15**, 230–8.

Wittich GR *et al.* (1992). Coaxial transthoracic fine-needle biopsy in patients with a history of malignant lymphoma. *Radiology* **183**,175–8.

Chapter 5

Psychosocial and spiritual dimensions of cancer pain

Jennifer Barraclough

Introduction

The psychosocial and spiritual dimensions of cancer pain are closely linked with the physical ones. Ideally, consideration of these aspects would be integrated with medical assessment and management for all patients from the time of their first presentation (Breitbart 1989, 1994; Breitbart & Payne 1998).

Many different, but overlapping, variables are relevant: mood, attitudes, understanding and expectations, communication with health care staff, personality, presence of psychiatric disorder, past illness experience, recent life events and difficulties, social network, cultural factors, religious and spiritual beliefs. In the late 1980s, Dalton (1988) suggested that only modest links between cancer pain and psychosocial variables had been demonstrated, with many aspects having received little systematic study. However, more recent reviews do indicate established links, with the need for a multidimensional model continuing to be stressed (Stiefel 1993).

Papers referenced in this chapter have been identified through searching the databases of Medline Express (1990–1/1999), Embase (1980–1/1999), PsychLIT (1988–98) and the Cochrane library (Issue 1, 1999), using combinations of the terms 'cancer pain', 'neoplasms', 'pain-psychology', 'religion and psychology', 'psychology', 'pain and coping' 'coping-behaviour' 'personality' and 'social-psychology'. This is not a systematic review as only those papers that appeared relevant from their titles and abstracts were examined in more detail. Many aspects of this complex topic do not readily lend themselves to a conventional evidence-based approach and, while hundreds of descriptive papers were found, there were few prospective studies of aetiology or randomised controlled trials of therapy.

Assessment and management will be considered in turn, drawing upon clinical experience as well as published studies.

Assessment

Definition

The Longman Dictionary of Contemporary English gives four definitions of pain and the first one is divided as follows:

> **1**. basic bodily sensation induced by injury, physical disorder, etc. and characterised by physical discomfort;
> **2**. acute mental or emotional distress or suffering: grief.

When patients say they are in pain, many health care professionals automatically assume they are talking about physical pain, but some are really using the second definition of the term.

Social/environmental settings

Cancer pain impairs activities of daily living, family and social life, hobbies and work (Strang 1992; Lancee *et al.* 1994). Conversely, the perceived severity of a pain may be affected by variations in day-to-day environment or social setting, being worse when patients feel lonely, bored, uncomfortable, too hot or too cold.

Relationship with psychological symptoms and psychiatric syndromes

Cross-sectional surveys of cancer patient populations show that pain is clearly associated with both psychological symptoms and psychiatric syndromes (Derogatis *et al.* 1983; Glover *et al.* 1995; Zimmerman *et al.* 1996). Depression, anxiety, and organic mental disorder are the most frequent syndromes both in cancer patient populations generally, and in cancer patients with pain. The relationship with depression (Spiegel *et al.* 1994) and anxiety (Velikova *et al.* 1995) has been specifically explored.

These associations may be explained in various ways. Poorly controlled pain has an impact on mood, often causing psychiatric symptoms of depression and anxiety, which resolve when adequate medical treatment is given. Less often, the opposite direction of causality predominates, and the pain is a symptom of a primary psychiatric syndrome, such as depressive illness (von Korff & Simon 1996), an anxiety state, or more global psychosocial distress, as in the phenomenon of 'somatisation'. Somatising patients may be having pain because of the physiological concomitants of anxiety, they may lack the vocabulary to articulate emotional issues, or they may be showing a 'social desirability' response influenced by the greater acceptability of physical complaints over psychological ones. Although such mechanisms undoubtedly contribute to complaints of pain among patients with cancer (Chaturvedi & Maguire 1998), some organic basis is usually present too, and the concept of somatisation must only be invoked with tact and care.

Most studies have been cross-sectional and therefore yield only limited information about the direction of causality. One prospective study (Syrjala & Chapko 1995) investigated psychosocial factors as predictors of pain from oral mucositis in 358 bone marrow transplant patients. While some psychosocial variables were significant predictors of pain in this sample, the effect was modest in comparison with biomedical variables. This particular type of pain provides a convenient model for research, but may have limited relevance to the pain of advanced cancer presenting in clinical practice.

Co-morbid severe mental health problems

Another aspect of this relationship is the assessment and management of pain for patients with whom communication is complicated by psychotic illness, learning difficulties or dementia, usually pre-dating their cancer. Such patients have often been excluded from palliative care and psycho-oncology research because of their advanced age, inability to consent and/or their place of care; however, their needs are currently being addressed (National Council for Hospice and Specialist Palliative Care Services 1999).

Desire for death

Suicide is up to twice as frequent among cancer patients as in the general population (Harris & Barraclough 1994), though seldom encountered by individual clinicians. Suicidal ideation and requests for euthanasia are much more common than completed suicide. Clinical depression is probably the main correlate of the desire to die (Chochinov *et al.* 1995), but pain is also a factor (Foley 1991) and was recorded in three-quarters of a series of cancer suicides (Heitanen *et al.* 1994).

Information and understanding about medical aspects

Certain beliefs in relation to cancer pain, which are prevalent among both patients and health care professionals (but not necessarily correct), seem likely to exacerbate its perceived severity. Examples include the assumption that dying from cancer inevitably means severe pain, or that all pains experienced by cancer patients result directly from the cancer and indicate cancer progression. Turk (1998) found cancer pain to be associated with more disability and less activity than non-cancer pain of comparable self-reported severity.

Prescribed medication

Other beliefs may be hampering the optimal use of effective therapies. Patients may take less than adequate doses of opioids because of reluctance to comply, fears about side-effects or the risk of addiction, a sense of stigma surrounding this class of drugs, mood disturbance or problems in communication with others (Ward *et al.* 1993; Glajchen *et al.* 1995). Less commonly, patients take excessive doses of prescribed drugs, or misuse 'unofficial' remedies, including alcohol (Bruera 1995) and cannabis. Regarding health care professionals, also, numerous barriers to the best use of medication exist (World Health Organization 1992). These include lack of scientific and clinical knowledge, restrictions on drug availability in certain countries, concerns about medico-legal aspects, and psychological attitudes, whether or not these are consciously recognised. Even those professionals who are highly skilled in the medical aspects of cancer pain management may have limited awareness of non-drug approaches (Zaza *et al.* 1999).

Some further points of peripheral relevance will be mentioned for completeness. Opioid analgesics may have psychiatric effects such as induction of cognitive impairment or delirium. Psychotropic drugs, including antidepressants, psychostimulants and antipsychotics, have a role in the adjuvant treatment of cancer pain (Twycross 1996). Complementary therapies such as acupuncture, aromatherapy and healing are used by approximately 20 per cent of cancer patients (Risberg *et al.* 1995), sometimes with the specific aim of pain relief.

Coping styles and attitudes to illness

This topic has attracted much research in medical psychology. As a broad simplification, coping styles can be divided into active coping as exemplified by the 'fighting spirit' response, and passive coping, as exemplified by 'hopelessness/helplessness'. The majority of studies have found that an active coping style is associated with less mental distress and better medical outcomes than a passive one, and many of the psychological interventions developed for cancer patients include, among their aims, the promotion of active coping styles. Clinically, however, it is important to respect individual ways of coping, and not impose the 'prison of positive thinking' in which excessive striving to fight the illness inhibits the processing of appropriate distress. Personality is likely to be an important variable but has received limited study in relation to cancer pain. There is a much larger literature on personality and chronic non-cancer pain (Asghari & Nicholas 1999).

Mental imagery

Some patients create visual representations of their pain, or other symptoms. This phenomenon can be used in therapy to explore attitudes towards pain, help ventilate emotions, and improve pain control through altering the image. A simple example would be changing the imagined colour of a pain from an angry red to a pale pink or blue, or changing the associated symbol from a savage tiger to a contented cat. This requires a relaxed state, and is sometimes done under hypnosis.

Personal meaning of illness

Lipowski (1970), writing about illness generally, listed the categories of: challenge, enemy, punishment, weakness, relief, strategy, irreparable loss and value. Descriptive applications of this model in relation to cancer pain are given by Barkwell (1991) and Ferrell & Dean (1995). Ersek & Ferrell (1994) provide a review.

Spiritual and religious aspects

Spiritual and religious aspects are concerned with the theme of personal meaning of pain at a deeper level, in relation to the meaning of the illness generally and to the value and purpose of life itself. There is no universal definition of spirituality, but it clearly relates to the non-material and includes concepts of meaning and purpose, and of the continuity and connectedness of life. This may be expressed through appreciation of nature or beauty, or through creativity, and does not necessarily involve religious faith or practice. Examples of the extensive literature in this field are referenced

(Derrickson 1996; Kearney 1996; Twycross 1996; *International Journal of Palliative Nursing* 1997; Howell 1998; Twycross 1999).

Sometimes this topic is considered within the context of specific religious faiths, or increasingly within a 'New Age' or 'holistic' framework. However, to list specific teachings on pain from specific religions would be an over-simplification. Some individuals' beliefs have practical implications for their pain management – for example, a reluctance to accept analgesic drugs could be rooted in the wish to take an attitude of detached meditative observation towards pain, a belief that it represents God's will, or the understanding of it as a 'karmic' phenomenon which needs to be experienced directly.

A strong spiritual or religious belief is sometimes associated with marked difficulties in coping with pain or terminal illness. Such difficulties could reflect a challenge to the faith of the individual concerned, their extremely high expectations of themselves, or their need to face their situation frankly without any recourse to denial.

Pain would sometimes appear to be an expression of spiritual distress, for patients who are tormented by an inability to find satisfactory answers to their existential dilemmas, which again illustrates that people may use the word 'pain' in different ways. This probably contributes to the syndromes known as 'overwhelming pain' and 'total pain', in which the different aspects of pain intertwine to cause severe acute distress.

Other patients find their faith becomes stronger during terminal illness and brings them great comfort. Others hope to find something worthwhile in their suffering.

Pearl

I will bear this pain
As the oyster its grain of sand
To make a pearl.

(Haiku quoted by courtesy of Camilla Connell)

Management

Good clinical practice

Skills in communication with patients and relatives, accepting psychosocial aspects as valid and non-stigmatised, and offering information about medical aspects are important in this field as in all clinical practice. Simple practical measures such as gentle exercise, listening to music or the presence of human or animal companionship (Phear 1996) may help. Such measures are often provided through home care or day-care programmes, the benefits of which often appear very obvious clinically, although less easy to validate through controlled trials (see, for example, Smeenk *et al.* 1998).

A review of the literature on more specific approaches follows.

Education about cancer pain

For staff, Breitbart *et al.* (1998) described favourable responses from 152 professionals who took part in the Network Project, a two-week observership at New York's Memorial Sloan-Kettering Cancer Center. This combined cancer pain management, psychosocial oncology and cancer rehabilitation. Follow-up of the participants showed their knowledge of these topics had improved, and that relevant educational activities in their own host institutions had increased.

For patients, also, descriptive studies give encouraging results. Ferrell *et al.* (1994) offered a pain education programme to elderly patients living at home. They found improved knowledge and more appropriate use of therapies, but did not demonstrate improved quality of life. De Wit *et al.* (1999) evaluated use of a pain diary for patients with chronic cancer pain following their discharge from hospital. Compliance was high and many of those who used the diary said it helped them to cope with the pain.

Less positive findings emerged from a large randomised controlled trial on inpatients with various 'high-mortality' medical diagnoses, including cancer (Desbiens *et al.* 1998). Their intervention comprised 'information, empowerment, advocacy, counselling and feedback' with patients, families and professional carers. The marginally better outcome in the treated group did not reach statistical significance and the authors concluded that 'patient empowerment and feedback did not decrease pain in seriously ill hospitalised adults.' However, this may have reflected barriers to delivering the intervention and the fact that it was offered so late in the illness, rather than ineffectiveness of its content.

Recognition and treatment of psychiatric disorder

The well-established associations between cancer pain and psychiatric disorder imply that some assessment of mood and mental state is appropriate for all cancer patients with pain. However, psychiatric disorders in cancer patients still often go undetected by oncologists, depression being especially easy to miss (Passik *et al.* 1998). As for how this situation can be improved, a simple question, 'Are you depressed?' (Chochinov 1995), or a visual analogue scale (Holland 1997) may be as good as more sophisticated screening questionnaires or interview techniques for the detection of depression.

The clinical management of psychiatric complications for cancer patients with pain has been thoroughly reviewed by Massie & Holland (1992). Although most clinical trials of psychological and psychiatric treatments have not included pain as a specific outcome measure, there is considerable evidence that psychological interventions for cancer patients are helpful for the treatment of anxiety and depression, and enhancement of quality of life (Fawzy *et al.* 1995; Meyer & Mark 1995). Psychotropic drugs have a role in selected cases (*Psycho-Oncology* 1998).

Psychological approaches to cancer pain

Of the many techniques included under this heading, the structured brief approaches now tend to be favoured over more traditional psychodynamic ones. However, different techniques suit different patients, and whatever technique is used, the quality of the therapeutic relationship is important. Cognitive behavioural therapy is designed to identify maladaptive patterns of thoughts and beliefs, examine their validity and experiment with alternatives, through collaboration between patient and therapist. Descriptive practical accounts of such an approach with cancer pain patients (Davis 1987; Golden & Gersh 1990; Loscalzo & Jacobsen 1990; Fishman 1992; Loscalzo 1996) emphasise the need for integration with medical care, as opposed to invoking psychological aspects as a 'last resort'. Other techniques include relaxation, hypnosis and imagery (Spiegel & Moore 1997; Wallace 1997), and creative therapies such as art (Connell 1998) and music (Beck 1991).

All these diverse approaches offer patients an enhanced sense of control and participation in their own treatment, and many are interesting and enjoyable in themselves. They can often be delivered in a small group setting. A majority of patients can probably benefit, whether or not they have identified psychological problems. The presence of severe emotional distress or psychiatric disorder does not necessarily contraindicate any of these therapies but does call for discretion.

Several controlled studies of psychological treatments have been carried out. A well-known trial of group therapy for patients with metastatic breast cancer (Spiegel & Bloom 1983) found that an intervention including hypnosis and group support achieved improved control of pain, among other benefits. Guided imagery significantly reduced post-operative pain, anxiety and analgesic requirements in a controlled study of patients undergoing primary surgery for bowel cancer (Tusek *et al.* 1997). Both guided imagery and progressive muscular relaxation appeared to provide effective pain relief for cancer patients in a military hospital (Graffam & Johnson 1987). Returning to the model of pain from oral mucositis following bone marrow transplantation, relaxation and imagery training were also found helpful in a controlled trial by Syrjala *et al.* (1995). Patients were randomised to four groups:

1. Treatment as usual
2. Therapist support
3. Relaxation and imagery training
4. Relaxation and imagery training plus training in cognitive behavioural coping skills.

Pain was measured by visual analogue scales. Groups 3 and 4 reported less pain than groups 1 and 2. Therapist support was not significantly better than treatment as usual; addition of cognitive behavioural therapy was not significantly more helpful than relaxation and imagery alone, which may be surprising in view of the established role of cognitive behavioural therapy in managing chronic non-cancer pain (Morley *et al.* 1999).

Conclusions

Psychological, social and spiritual aspects of cancer pain have received limited systematic study, and the evidence-based approach is only partly appropriate to this topic. Although medical diagnosis and treatment hold centre stage for most cases, this broader supporting perspective is always important, and it is desirable to aim for an integrated approach to assessment and management. This may well be rewarded by greater patient and staff satisfaction and possibly, though this is yet to be established, reduced costs on medical care.

Acknowledgements

The author wishes to thank: David Hardy, Clare Harris, Meg Roberts, Victoria Slater, Ben Steinberg and Phil Wiffen.

References

Asghari MA & Nicholas MK (1999). Personality and adjustment to chronic pain. *Pain Reviews* **6**, 85–97.

Barkwell DP (1991). Ascribed meaning: a critical factor in coping and pain attenuation in patients with cancer-related pain. *Journal of Palliative Care* **7**, 5–14.

Beck SL (1991). The therapeutic use of music for cancer-related pain. *Oncology Nursing Forum* **18**, 1327–37.

Breitbart W (1989). Psychiatric management of cancer pain. *Cancer* **63**, 2336–42.

Breitbart W (1994). Cancer pain management guidelines: implications for psycho-oncology. *Psycho-Oncology* **3**, 103–8.

Breitbart W & Payne DK (1998). Pain. In *Psycho-Oncology* (ed. J Holland), pp.450–67. Oxford University Press, New York, USA.

Breitbart W *et al.* (1998). The Network project: a multidisciplinary cancer education and training program in pain management, rehabilitation and psychosocial issues. *Journal of Pain and Symptom Management* **15**, 18–26.

Bruera E *et al.* (1995). The frequency of alcoholism among patients with pain due to terminal cancer. *Journal of Pain and Symptom Management* **10**, 599–603.

Chaturvedi SK & Maguire GP (1998). Persistent somatization in cancer: a controlled follow-up study. *Journal of Psychosomatic Research* **45**, 249–56.

Chochinov HM *et al.* (1995). Desire for death in the terminally ill. *American Journal of Psychiatry* **152**, 1185–91.

Chochinov HM *et al.* (1997). 'Are you depressed?' Screening for depression in the terminally ill. *American Journal of Psychiatry* **154**, 674–6.

Connell C (1998). *Something understood: art therapy in cancer care.* Wrexham Publications, London.

Dalton JA & Feuerstein M (1988). Biobehavioural factors in cancer pain. *Pain* **33**, 137–47.

Davis M *et al.* (1987). Behavioural interventions in coping with cancer-related pain. *British Journal of Guidance and Counselling* **15**, 17–28.

De Wit R *et al.* (1999). Evaluation of the use of a pain diary in chronic cancer pain patients at home. *Pain* **79**, 89–99.

Derogatis L *et al.* (1983). The prevalence of psychiatric disorders among cancer patients. *Journal of the American Medical Association* **249**, 751–7.

Derrickson BS (1996). The spiritual work of the dying: a framework and case studies. *Hospice Journal* **11**, 11–30.

Desbiens NA *et al.* (1998). Patient empowerment and feedback did not decrease pain in seriously ill hospitalised adults. *Pain* **75**, 237–46.

Ersek M & Ferrell BR (1994). Providing relief from cancer pain by assisting in the search for meaning. *Journal of Palliative Care* **10**, 15–22.

Fawzy IF *et al.* (1995). Critical review of psychosocial interventions in cancer care. *Archives of General Psychiatry* **52**, 100–13.

Ferrell BR *et al.* (1994). Pain management for elderly patients with cancer at home. *Cancer* **74**, 2139–46.

Ferrell BR & Dean G (1995). The meaning of cancer pain. *Seminars in Oncology Nursing* **11**, 17–22.

Fishman B (1992). The cognitive behavioural perspective on pain management in terminal illness. *Hospice Journal* **8**, 73–88.

Foley KM (1991). The relationship of pain and symptom management to patient requests for physician-assisted suicide. *Journal of Pain and Symptom Management* **6**, 289–97.

Glajchen M *et al.* (1995). Psychosocial barriers to cancer pain relief. *Cancer Practitioner* **3**, 76–82.

Glover J *et al.* (1995). Mood states of oncology outpatients: does pain make a difference? *Journal of Pain and Symptom Management* **10**, 120–8.

Graffam S & Johnson A (1987). A comparison of two relaxation strategies for the relief of pain and its distress. *Journal of Pain and Symptom Management* **2**, 229–31.

Harris EC & Barraclough BM (1994). Suicide as an outcome for medical disorders. *Medicine* **73**, 281–96.

Hietanen P *et al.* (1994). Do cancer suicides differ from others? *Psycho-Oncology* **3**, 189–96.

Holland JC (1997). Preliminary guidelines for the treatment of distress. *Oncology* **11**, 109–17.

Howell D (1998). Reaching to the depths of the soul: understanding and exploring meaning in illness. *Can Oncol Nurs J* **8**, 12–23.

International Journal of Palliative Nursing (1997). **3** (Issue devoted to spiritual care).

Kearney M (1996). *Mortally wounded.* Marino Books, Dublin, Ireland.

Lancee WJ *et al.* (1994). The impact of pain and impaired role performance on distress in patients with cancer. *Canadian Journal of Psychiatry* **39**, 617–22.

Lipowski Z (1970). Physical illness, the individual and the coping process. *Psychiatric Medicine* **1**, 91–102.

Loscalzo M (1996). Psychological approaches to the management of pain in patients with advanced cancer. *Haematology Oncology Clinics of North America* **10**, 139–55.

Loscalzo M & Jacobsen PB (1990). Practical behavioural approaches to the effective management of pain and distress. *Journal of Psychosocial Oncology* **8**, 139–69.

Massie MJ & Holland JC (1992). The cancer patient with pain: psychiatric complications and their management. *Journal of Pain and Symptom Management* **7**, 99–109.

Meyer TJ & Mark MM (1995). Effects of psychosocial intervention with adult cancer patients: a meta-analysis of randomised experiments. *Health Psychology* **14**, 101–8.

Morley S *et al.* (1999). Systematic review and meta-analysis of randomized controlled trials of chronic behaviour therapy and behaviour therapy for chronic pain in adults, excluding headache. *Pain* **80**, 1–13.

National Council for Hospice and Specialist Palliative Care Services and Scottish Partnership Agency for Palliative and Cancer Care (1999). *Palliative care for adults with mental health problems: a qualitative needs assessment* (in preparation).

Passik SD *et al.* (1998). Oncologists' recognition of depression in their patients with cancer. *Journal of Clinical Oncology* **16**, 1594–600.

Phear DN (1996). A study of animal companionship in a day hospice. *Palliative Medicine* **10**, 336–8.

Psycho-Oncology (1998). **7**(4) (Special issue on psychopharmacology in cancer medicine).

Risberg T *et al.* (1995). The use of non-proven therapy among patients treated in Norwegian oncological departments. A cross-sectional national multicentre study. *European Journal of Cancer* **31**A, 1785–9.

Smeenk FWJM *et al.* (1998). Effectiveness of home care programmes for patients with incurable cancer on their quality of life and time spent in hospital: systematic review. *BMJ* **316**, 1939–44.

Spiegel D *et al.* (1994). Pain and depression in patients with cancer. *Cancer* **74**, 2570–8.

Spiegel D & Bloom JR (1983). Group therapy and hypnosis reduce metastatic breast carcinoma pain. *Psychosomatic Medicine* **4**, 333–9.

Spiegel D & Moore R (1997). Imagery and hypnosis in the treatment of cancer patients. *Oncology-Huntingt* **11**, 1179–89; discussion 1189–95.

Stiefel F (1993). Psychosocial aspects of cancer pain. *Supportive Care and Cancer* **1**, 130–4.

Strang P (1992). Emotional and social aspects of cancer pain. *Acta Oncologica* **31**, 323–6.

Syrjala KL *et al.* (1995). Relaxation and imagery and cognitive-behavioural training reduce pain during cancer treatment: a controlled clinical trial. *Pain* **63**, 189–98.

Syrjala KL & Chapko ME (1995). Evidence for a biopsychosocial model of cancer treatment-related pain. *Pain* **61**, 69–79.

Turk DC *et al.* (1998). Adaptation to metastatic cancer pain, regional/local cancer pain and non-cancer pain: role of psychological and behavioural factors. *Pain* **74**, 247–56.

Tusek DL *et al.* (1997). Guided imagery: a significant advance in the care of patients undergoing elective colorectal surgery. *Diseases of Colon and Rectum* **40**, 172–8.

Twycross RG (1996). *Pain relief in advanced cancer*. Churchill Livingstone, Edinburgh.

Twycross RG (1999). Pain and suffering. In *Introducing palliative care*. Radcliffe Medical Press, Oxford.

Velikova G *et al.* (1995). The relationship of cancer pain to anxiety. *Psychotherapeutics and Psychosomatics* **63**, 181–4.

von Korff M & Simon G (1996). The relationship between pain and depression. *British Journal of Psychiatry* **168**(Suppl.30), 101–8.

Wallace KG (1997). Analysis of recent literature concerning relaxation and imagery interventions for cancer pain. *Cancer Nursing* **20**, 79–87.

Ward SE *et al.* (1993). Patient-related barriers to management of cancer pain. *Pain* **52**, 319–24.

World Health Organization Expert Committee on Cancer Pain Relief and Active Supportive Care (1992). Pain control. Barriers to the use of available information. *Cancer* **70**(Suppl.), 1438–49.

Zaza C *et al.* (1999). Health care professionals' familiarity with non-pharmacological strategies for managing cancer pain. *Psycho-Oncology* **8**, 99–111.

Zimmerman L *et al.* (1996). Psychological variables and cancer pain. *Cancer Nursing* **19**, 44–53.

PART 2

Evidence and treatment

Chapter 6

Agreeing a gold standard in the management of cancer pain: the role of opioids

Geoffrey W Hanks and Colette Hawkins

Introduction

Most pain in cancer responds to pharmacological treatment using orally administered analgesics and adjuvants. Current management is based on the World Health Organization's (WHO) concept of an 'analgesic ladder', which involves a simple stepwise approach to the use of analgesic drugs and is essentially a framework of principles rather than a rigid protocol (Table 6.1). This allows considerable flexibility in the choice of specific drugs, and should be regarded as but one part of a comprehensive strategy for managing cancer pain. Symptomatic drug treatment is used in an integrated way with disease-modifying therapy and non-drug measures.

Criticism from a systematic review (Jadad & Browman 1995) of the strength of the evidence to support the use of the WHO method is misplaced. Criticism of the WHO validation studies centres on the lack of randomised controlled trials (RCTs), the retrospective nature of some of the studies, short follow-up, high withdrawal rates and poorly defined outcome measures. A more pragmatic view would take into account the large number of patients involved (almost 4,000), the remarkably consistent results in different countries and environments (Table 6.2), the weight of supporting anecdotal clinical experience over the last three decades and the impossibility of conducting RCTs now that the WHO method is a world standard.

The most important part of the WHO method, and the reason for its success, is the use of oral opioids for moderate-to-severe pain. Until now morphine has been the benchmark 'step 3' opioid because it is effective and familiar to prescribing

Table 6.1 The WHO method for cancer pain relief: the principles

Simplicity – in choice of analgesics
Simplicity – in choice of route (oral)
Individualisation of dose, particularly of strong opioids
Continuous pain requires continuous medication
Use of adjuvant analgesics
Treatment of adverse effects to allow adequate dose titration

Table 6.2 The WHO method for cancer pain relief: validation studies

Authors	n	Adequate analgesia (%)
Ventafridda *et al.* (1987)	1,229	71
Walker *et al.* (1988)	13	69
Goisis *et al.* (1989)	45	93
Ventafridda *et al.* (1990)	261	76
Takeda *et al.* (1990)	205	97
Wenk *et al.* (1991)	28	100
Siguan *et al.* (1992)	86	86
Zech *et al.* (1995)	2,118	88
	3,985	**mean 85**

physicians and is the oldest, cheapest and most widely available of this group of drugs. However, in recent years a number of alternatives to morphine have been introduced in different countries and it is appropriate now to appraise the evidence relating to the clinical use of these drugs to see whether it is possible to establish a hierarchy which should influence prescribing.

We should draw attention at the outset to the paucity of RCTs in this area. One reason is that many of the most important drugs have been in clinical use for a very long time and were introduced without the requirements of proof of efficacy that apply today. Patients with chronic cancer pain needing regular opioids are also a particularly difficult group to study and there are major problems with recruitment to trials and attrition. RCTs are difficult in such circumstances but not impossible and more attention is now given to robust trial methodology in the evaluation of new drugs or new formulations of old ones.

Morphine in cancer pain

In the treatment of chronic cancer pain morphine is given by mouth, the dose is titrated upwards to achieve adequate relief and there is no arbitrary maximum; doses are given regularly to prevent recurrence of pain; and common side-effects such as nausea and constipation are treated to allow dose titration and maintenance. In order to capitalise on the flexibility of this drug, both normal-release and modified-release formulations are required (Hanks *et al.* 1996) and a range of oral dosage forms are now available (normal-release solutions and tablets, and 12- and 24-hour modified-release tablets or capsules). Paradoxically, there are still many countries where it is easier to prescribe a modified-release preparation than normal-release (in Italy, for example), and more importantly there are still many parts of the world where the drug is extremely difficult to prescribe at all (for example, India and the developing world in general).

Pharmacokinetics

The pharmacokinetics of morphine have been accurately described only relatively recently (Hoskin & Hanks 1990; Glare & Walsh 1991), partly because many studies carried out before the mid-1980s produced spurious results from the unwitting use of cross-reacting assay methods. Morphine is almost completely absorbed when given by mouth but undergoes extensive first-pass metabolism so that its systemic availability is only 20–30 per cent (Hoskin *et al.* 1989) (with wide inter-individual variation). About 90 per cent is converted to metabolites: mainly morphine-3-glucuronide (M3G) and morphine-6-glucuronide (M6G), and to a much lesser extent normorphine, codeine, morphine ethereal sulphate and others (Yeh *et al.* 1977). The relative amounts of the glucuronide metabolites vary considerably between individuals and quite different figures are reported in different studies. It is clear that M3G is the major metabolite but a recent systematic review (Faura *et al.* 1998) describes a wide range of ratios of the glucuronide metabolites to morphine in different studies (0.001–504 for M3G : M, and 0–97 for M6G : M) . This is one reason for the confusion about the role of the metabolites of morphine. Quite different interpretations and conclusions have been reached by different investigators because the data have varied so much from study to study.

M6G binds to µ receptors and has potent analgesic activity (Shimomura *et al.* 1971) and probably contributes to the pharmacological effect of repeated-dose oral morphine (Hanks *et al.* 1987), although its precise role and the magnitude of its contribution remain unclear. M6G is excreted in the urine with an elimination half-life of 2–3 hours. In patients with renal impairment M6G accumulates and, as glomerular filtration rate deteriorates, its half-life progressively lengthens. This almost certainly accounts for the toxic effects of morphine in this situation (Osborne *et al.* 1986) and means that caution is required when using morphine in patients with renal failure.

The role of M3G is even less clear. M3G has long been thought to be inert but recent data indicate that, when injected directly into the subarachnoid space or into the cerebral ventricles of rats, it causes hyperalgesia, motor excitation and respiratory stimulation. M3G also appears to antagonise the analgesic effects of morphine and M6G in some animal models. However, there are no reliable data to support these effects in humans and M3G does not bind to opioid receptors (Shimomura *et al.* 1971; Bartlett & Smith 1995), so if it is responsible for neurotoxic adverse effects in humans, it does so through some non-opioid mechanism. At present this is speculative and on the basis of the available evidence it remains an open question as to whether M3G is responsible for any of the CNS toxicity of morphine.

Normorphine, codeine and other 6-substituted metabolites of morphine and codeine are active µ agonists (and normorphine has affinity for δ receptors too) but these metabolites are produced in insignificant amounts and are not likely to have any clinical relevance. However, there is a potential here for some contribution to pharmacodynamic or toxic effects if any situation arises which increases the relative amounts of these active metabolites.

Pharmacology and clinical efficacy

Morphine is the prototype μ agonist (with some effects also at κ and δ receptors) and is the standard opioid for severe pain against which others are measured. However, there is a dearth of RCT efficacy data to support the use of repeated-dose oral morphine. Most of the available RCTs involve comparisons of normal-release formulations with 12- or 24-hour controlled-release preparations (Hanks 1990). These studies were designed to prove equivalence of the modified-release preparation and most involve small numbers of patients studied for short periods of time. There are substantial anecdotal experience and descriptive data which demonstrate the effectiveness of oral morphine in cancer pain but the relative lack of high-quality clinical trials is reflected in some of the current controversies relating to the way in which we use this and similar drugs in cancer pain. There is much opinion (often divergent) but limited hard evidence.

Opioid responsiveness and adverse effects

Morphine appears to have no clinically relevant ceiling effect to analgesia. Doses of oral morphine may vary 1,000-fold in different patients to achieve the same endpoint of pain relief. Morphine probably has the widest dose range of any drug used in modern therapeutics. As the dose is increased, analgesic effects increase as a log-linear function until either pain relief is achieved or adverse effects supervene. In this case higher doses could theoretically produce greater analgesia but dose escalation is not possible because of unwanted effects (which effectively defines the 'responsiveness' of the pain in that particular patient).

Morphine is not the panacea for cancer pain and a new jargon has developed around the clinical situations where morphine does not produce straightforward pain relief, or where unwanted effects prevent its optimal use. It has become clear, for example, that some types of pain do not respond well or fully to morphine. This is rarely an all-or-none phenomenon, so terms such as 'opioid-resistant' are inaccurate and it is preferable to describe such pain as 'poorly responsive' (Hanks & Forbes 1997). Neuropathic pain is the commonest example. It has been suggested that pain sensitivity and response to opioid analgesics may be genetically determined at least in part. By manipulating the gene for the μ receptor, mice can be made to express fewer receptors, are more sensitive to pain and require larger doses of morphine to relieve it (Uhl et al. 1999).

Other situations where oral morphine is not ideal include the management of acute exacerbations of pain or acute episodic pain. Pain on weight-bearing or movement (so-called incident pain), for example, can be difficult to control because if the regular background analgesia is titrated sufficiently to cover the movement-related exacerbations, it is too much for the patient at rest and will cause excessive adverse effects. This is because there is generally a balance between pain and the CNS-depressant effects of opioids: when there is no painful stimulus, CNS effects are more prominent. The use of normal-release 'breakthrough' doses of opioid in this situation is often unsatisfactory because pain relief is not obtained quickly enough and the effect of an extra dose may then be merely to cause increased sedation over the next few hours.

CNS adverse effects are the most likely to limit dose escalation. Fears about respiratory depression and 'addiction' have proved unfounded and these potential problems do not complicate the use of morphine in chronic cancer pain. Nausea and vomiting may occur but invariably resolve within a few days, as does drowsiness and sedation. The main continuing adverse effect which requires ongoing vigilance and treatment is constipation.

Opioid-switching/rotation

In recent years attention has focused on possible toxic effects of morphine metabolites in frail patients who may be dehydrated, with borderline renal insufficiency. It has been postulated that patients may become obtunded as a result of the accumulation of toxic metabolites and this results in poor fluid intake and further dehydration and toxicity. Such patients may have intolerable adverse effects with morphine, while achieving inadequate analgesia. The incidence of the problem and the suggested pathophysiology have been the subject of some controversy (de Stoutz *et al.* 1995; Fainsinger & Toro 1998; Hawley *et al.* 1998).

It has long been observed anecdotally that in patients experiencing severe adverse effects with morphine, switching to an alternative agonist may allow titration to adequate analgesia without the same disabling effects. The explanation is not clear but it is probably partly related to the fact that there is incomplete cross-tolerance between the commonly available opioid agonists. There are also some differences between the drugs in their affinity for different opioid receptors, different types of pain may respond differentially to different opioids because of this, and active metabolites may be implicated. In some centres it has been found necessary or beneficial to change to an alternative opioid in up to 40 per cent of patients with pain associated with advanced cancer (de Stoutz *et al.* 1995). Sometimes several changes of drug are employed in the same patient and the term 'opioid-rotation' has been coined to describe this practice. Our experience has been different: we would expect to run into problems in perhaps 2–3 per cent of patients receiving regular oral morphine and in some of these patients resolution of the adverse effects, while maintaining adequate analgesia, can be achieved by reducing the dose of the opioid. However, in some cases a substitution may be necessary and effective.

There are no RCT data to establish which practice is right (or whether either is legitimate) and whether switching between opioids should be encouraged more often where it is rarely done and less often where it is done frequently. There are some clues as to why the reported incidence of morphine toxicity varies so greatly: higher doses of morphine or other opioids and less frequent use of adjuvants may result in more problems with the opioid, and this would encourage a change of opioid. The availability of effective alternatives to morphine is also an important determinant of the frequency with which changes in opioids are made. Not surprisingly the practice is more common where there is a greater choice of drugs. This is an area where well-designed RCTs would help to define best practice. Clearly, opioid rotation complicates pain management and this is a disadvantage for non-specialists. However, it may be a relatively simple strategy (for specialists) which could reap useful rewards in patients who are not doing well with their first-line drugs.

When a patient is experiencing intractable adverse effects despite routine measures to control them, there are two potential strategies which may improve the situation: administration of an alternative opioid agonist, as discussed above, or administration of the same opioid by another route.

As far as different routes are concerned, most debate has focused on the utility of spinal (epidural and intrathecal) administration of opioids. If a patient has a demonstrably opioid-responsive pain but develops severe adverse effects with systemic administration, it may be worthwhile considering spinal administration of an opioid, either alone or in conjunction with a local anaesthetic or other agent such as clonidine.

Morphine: summary

Morphine is effective, flexible and does not appear to have a clinical relevant ceiling dose. It has been the most widely available of the strong opioids in a range of oral formulations and there is substantial clinical experience with morphine, not just in the management of cancer pain. Its limitations include: poor systemic availability by the oral route, which influences the speed of onset of action and also contributes to the great variability between patients in terms of dose requirements and response; and active metabolites which may be responsible for toxicity particularly in patients with renal impairment. In addition, some types of pain respond poorly to morphine.

Alternatives to morphine

Recent years have seen a number of alternatives to morphine being advocated, either new molecules or novel formulations of existing, and sometimes very old, drugs. There are few RCTs involving head-to-head comparisons of alternative opioids and this is an important gap that needs to be filled. However, there are well-described differences between these drugs in pharmacological and pharmacokinetic profiles and this evidence is reviewed below.

Methadone

Methadone is a synthetic opioid introduced in the 1950s, which has been used both as a first-line drug in the treatment of cancer pain and also as an alternative to morphine. It is widely available in oral formulations and is cheap, but it is complicated to use because of the pronounced inter-individual variability in its pharmacokinetics and dynamics.

Pharmacokinetics

Methadone is rapidly absorbed after oral administration and has a bioavailability of about 80 per cent. Its plasma half-life is long, averaging approximately 24 hours (with a range of 17 to over 100 hours) and the drug accumulates on chronic dosing (Inturrisi & Verebely 1972; Verebely *et al.* 1975). There is great variation between patients in pharmacokinetic parameters. Methadone is extensively distributed and bound to tissue proteins with slow transfer between these tissue stores and plasma and this contributes to the long half-life. The major metabolic pathway is by demethylation and the metabolites are inactive (Pohland *et al.* 1971).

Pharmacology and clinical efficacy

Methadone has both μ and δ receptor effects and the recent resurgence of interest in this drug has been stimulated by its putative N-methyl-D-aspartate (NMDA) blocking effects (Gorman *et al.* 1997), and thus its potential for greater efficacy in neuropathic pain and other difficult pain problems. However, there are at present no clinical trial data to support any suggestion that methadone is more effective than other opioids in these difficult pain problems.

The major drawbacks of methadone in clinical practice are the discrepancy between the duration of its initial analgesic effect and plasma elimination half-life, and the inter-individual variation in kinetics and dynamics. In single-dose studies methadone is only marginally more potent than morphine. However, with repeated administration it is several times more potent (Ventafridda *et al.* 1986), and its duration of action is also longer. Most patients initially require doses at 4–6 hourly intervals to maintain analgesia (Grochow *et al.* 1989), but the frequency of dosing must gradually be decreased to once or twice a day. The need for more frequent dosing at the initiation of treatment or when the dose is changed puts patients at risk of drug accumulation with consequent sedation, confusion and even death (Ettinger *et al.* 1979). The difficulties of determining an equianalgesic dose of methadone when changing from another opioid have also been recently highlighted (Ripamonti *et al.* 1998). Methadone requires careful tailoring to individual patients: published tables of equianalgesic doses may be quite misleading.

Methadone is an effective analgesic in cancer pain although there are limited published clinical data (Fainsinger *et al.* 1993). Its potential advantages over morphine are its rapid absorption and onset of action, its greater bioavailability and long duration of action, and its low cost. Methadone may also have some advantage related to its putative NMDA receptor-blocking effect, although this remains theoretical at present. Against these potential advantages must be set the major disadvantages related to the complexity of its pharmacokinetics and the great variability between patients in both its pharmacokinetics and pharmacodynamic effects. This makes the drug difficult to use in clinical practice and rules it out as a first-line option in cancer pain management. It will continue to have a place as an alternative to morphine but is not recommended to non-specialists.

Hydromorphone

Hydromorphone is a semi-synthetic congener of morphine and a potent μ agonist. Originally synthesised in the 1920s and used as an antitussive for patients with tuberculosis, it is now established as a potent analgesic. In the USA hydromorphone was more widely used than morphine for cancer pain, until the introduction of modified-release morphine sulphate in the late 1980s. Hydromorphone can be given by oral, rectal, parenteral and spinal routes, although there is no injectable formulation currently available in the UK.

Pharmacokinetics

The completeness of absorption of hydromorphone from the gastrointestinal tract varies widely between individuals and the drug undergoes extensive first-pass metabolism resulting in a systemic availability variously reported to be 37–62 per cent (Vallner *et al.* 1981; Inturrisi *et al.* 1988). The elimination half-life is 1.5-3 hours, and most of the drug is excreted as glucuronide conjugates. Metabolism takes place in the liver, mainly to hydromorphone-3-glucuronide (H3G). Two minor metabolites, dihydromorphine and dihydroisomorphine, have been shown to be pharmacologically active in animal models but they are produced in very small amounts (Cone *et al.* 1977). H3G is excreted in the urine and accumulates in renal failure (Babul *et al.* 1995), and there has been speculation that this metabolite (and perhaps others) contribute to the neuroexcitatory toxicity that has been reported in some patients receiving high doses of hydromorphone, and also described in patients with renal failure receiving the drug. However, while there are pharmacokinetic data which confirm that H3G accumulates in renal failure, there is really no good evidence that it is pharmacologically active. On the other hand, the 6-hydroxy metabolites (dihydromorphine and dihydroisomorphine) are active but are produced in insignificant amounts in normal circumstances and there is no direct evidence that they accumulate in renal failure. This is of relevance to patients with renal impairment who may develop toxicity with usual doses of morphine. The available data are inconclusive but a trial of hydromorphone in patients experiencing major problems with morphine in this situation seems reasonable. However, it may well prove to be the case that a reduction in dose or dosing interval may also be necessary with hydromorphone in patients with renal impairment.

Pharmacology and clinical efficacy

Hydromorphone is a μ selective agonist similar to morphine, with weak affinity for κ and δ receptors. Single-dose studies have shown that it is between 5 and 10 times as potent as morphine (Houde 1986), and a ratio of 7.5:1 has been recommended in the repeated-dose setting in the UK (McDonald & Miller 1997). The oral-to-parenteral potency ratio (again derived from single-dose studies) is 1:5 (Houde 1986). An important advantage of hydromorphone is that it is much more soluble than morphine so that high doses require only small volumes for injection. Unfortunately, this advantage is negated in the UK where no parenteral formulation is available.

Hydromorphone is an effective, potent opioid analgesic, but, as with morphine, there is a relative lack of RCT data, particularly in chronic cancer pain. There are some recent studies which demonstrate that normal-release and controlled-release formulations of hydromorphone are equivalent in terms of pain relief and side-effects (Hays *et al.* 1994; Bruera *et al.* 1996). The available information suggests that its efficacy and adverse-effect profile is similar to morphine (except when given by the epidural route when hydromorphone seems much less likely to cause pruritus) (Chaplan *et al.* 1992).

The potential advantages of hydromorphone are its potency and a possibly better pharmacokinetic profile in patients with renal impairment (although this may prove not to be the case). Limitations to its use in the UK are its lack of familiarity to physicians, confusion about its relative potency, less flexibility in terms of available oral dose units, and the lack of a parenteral formulation. While hydromorphone is increasingly employed as an alternative to morphine, the overall use of this drug remains low in the UK.

Fentanyl

Fentanyl is a semi-synthetic opioid and an established intravenous anaesthetic and analgesic drug, which is about 80 times as potent as parenteral morphine. Until recently, it was only used by intravenous injection or infusion and was rarely employed in the management of cancer pain. However, fentanyl is now available in two novel formulations – transdermal and oral transmucosal – and both have applications in cancer pain. The pharmacokinetics of fentanyl are a function of the route of administration, and these two formulations produce quite different kinetic and dynamic profiles.

Pharmacology

Fentanyl is a highly selective μ agonist (Yeadon & Kitchen 1988). It appears to be associated with less tendency to cause histamine release (Rosow *et al.* 1982) and seems to have less effect on gastrointestinal transit time (Megens *et al.* 1998). There is accumulating evidence that when used for chronic cancer pain, fentanyl causes less constipation than morphine.

Pharmacokinetics: intravenous administration

When given intravenously, systemic clearance occurs in two phases, the first related to rapid redistribution of the drug into body tissues and the other due to hepatic and renal drug elimination (Mather 1983) (Figure 6.1). Fentanyl is highly lipophilic and within minutes of an intravenous (IV) injection is rapidly taken up by body tissues (Hess *et al.* 1972); its terminal elimination half-life has been variously reported between 2 and 10 hours. Metabolism occurs in the liver to norfentanyl and the lesser metabolites 4-N-anilino piperidine and hydroxy (phenyl) fentanyl (McClain & Hug 1980). The metabolites are inactive. When used intravenously, fentanyl has a very short duration of action of 0.5–1 hour. This is related to the rapid redistribution of the drug rather than to elimination.

Transdermal fentanyl

The use of fentanyl for cancer pain followed the development of new formulations, the first being the transdermal therapeutic system (TTS-fentanyl), which has enabled topical delivery of the drug. The low molecular weight and high lipid solubility of fentanyl facilitate absorption through the skin. The delivery system is in the form of a 'patch' which comprises four layers: a backing polyester film, the drug layer in gel form, a copolymer membrane controlling the rate of drug delivery, and a silicone adhesive (Lehmann & Zech 1992). The adhesive layer is saturated with fentanyl and

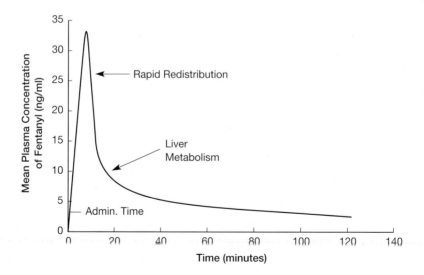

Source: Fine (1997) (Reproduced with permission)

Figure 6.1 Blood levels of fentanyl after IV administration. Systemic clearance occurs in two general phases, one related to redistribution of the drug into body tissues and the other due to hepatic and renal drug elimination

delivers an initial bolus on application of the patch (Lehmann & Zech 1992). The copolymer membrane releases fentanyl at a constant rate of 25 µg/hr per 10 cm^2. Patches are available in four dose strengths from 25 µg/hr to 100 µg/hr, with dose delivered being proportional to the surface area of the patch. Each patch is designed to deliver the drug over a three-day period.

Pharmacokinetics

Fentanyl is undetectable in the systemic circulation for 1–2 hours after application of the patch (Varvel *et al.* 1989; Lehmann & Zech 1992). Serum levels then rise, with analgesic effects evident within 8–16 hours and steady state is achieved prior to the second dose at 72 hours (Portenoy *et al.* 1993). Following removal of the patch, serum levels drop to 50 per cent by about 17 hours (Varvel *et al.* 1989). This is significantly longer than the terminal half-life of intravenous fentanyl, indicating the development of a subcutaneous depot of active drug. The pharmacokinetics of TTS- fentanyl show wide variability between patients (Portenoy *et al.* 1993) and some patients require a patch change every 48 hours rather than the recommended 72 hours (Yeo *et al.* 1997; Donner *et al.* 1998). There is no evidence of metabolism within the skin.

Clinical efficacy

Open clinical trials of TTS-fentanyl have demonstrated that it is effective and well tolerated in the management of cancer pain (Donner *et al.* 1996; Ahmedzai & Brooks 1997; Grond *et al.* 1997; Sloan *et al.* 1998). It may be particularly useful in patients unable to take oral medication (Grond *et al.* 1997). However, the pharmacokinetics of the drug administered in this way make it generally less flexible than shorter-acting preparations. While the three-day duration of action is an important advantage for patients with stable opioid requirements, it can complicate management of patients with unstable pain whose opioid requirements are fluctuating. The subcutaneous depot adds to this difficulty when patients' pain goes suddenly out of control, in terms of causing some uncertainty in selecting appropriate doses of alternative short-acting opioids which may be required to regain control of the situation.

There has been some controversy too about the equianalgesic dose ratio of fentanyl when administered transdermally, and the appropriate starting dose (Hanks & Fallon 1995; Storey 1995; Donner *et al.* 1996). It seems sensible to be conservative when initiating treatment with TTS-fentanyl. The lag time before analgesic plasma concentrations are achieved (12–16 hours) means that patients need a short-acting opioid to 'top-up' with and this should cope also with any relative underdosing. Thus the conversion ratio and starting doses recommended by the manufacturers seem appropriate.

There is both experimental and clinical evidence that TTS-fentanyl is associated with less constipation than morphine (Ahmedzai & Brooks 1997; Megens *et al.* 1998; Haazen *et al.* 1999). This seems to be a function of the much greater lipophilicity of fentanyl and its rapid passage across the blood brain barrier. As a result, low doses are required to produce analgesia and these have minimal effects on the gastrointestinal tract. In contrast analgesia with morphine is only achieved at doses which have marked effects on the gastrointestinal tract.

Other reports of less side-effects (nausea, vomiting, drowsiness) with TTS-fentanyl are difficult to evaluate in the absence of double-blind RCTs. Skin irritation (mostly mild erythema) has been reported with an incidence of up to 13 per cent (Donner et al. 1996). This does not usually limit use of the patch. Conversion from morphine to TTS-fentanyl occasionally precipitates a morphine-withdrawal syndrome (Zenz et al. 1994). This typically occurs within 24 hours of discontinuing morphine and is characterised by 'flu-like' symptoms, abdominal cramps, diarrhoea, anxiety and agitation. It is difficult to be certain what is the underlying mechanism here, and the incidence is unclear. However, all patients converted from morphine to TTS-fentanyl should have access to normal-release morphine preparations to manage transient withdrawal symptoms.

TTS-fentanyl in thus effective and well tolerated but best reserved for patients with stable opioid requirements. In such patients it works well and has high patient acceptability. It may cause less constipation than morphine. Its long duration of action (and prolonged elimination half-life) may be a disadvantage in patients with fluctuating pain, or when pain goes out of control. It will not be, therefore, the first-line choice for all patients.

Oral transmucosal fentanyl citrate

Oral transmucosal fentanyl citrate (OTFC) is a novel non-invasive dosage form of fentanyl that has been licensed in the USA both as an anaesthetic pre-medication for children and adults, and as a treatment for acute episodic ('breakthrough') pain in cancer patients maintained on opioid analgesics. OTFC units consist of a fentanyl-impregnated sweetened and hardened lozenge on a plastic handle. The lozenge is applied against the buccal mucosa and as it dissolves in saliva a proportion of the drug diffuses across the oral mucosa. The rest is swallowed and partially absorbed in the stomach and intestine. OTFC is available in a range of dosage units containing 200–1600 µg fentanyl.

Pharmacokinetics

Transmucosal absorption into the blood stream is rapid with peak plasma concentrations achieved at 20 minutes and a bioavailability of about 50 per cent (Streisand et al 1991) (Table 6.3). It seems that approximately half of the bioavailable drug is absorbed through the buccal mucosa, where it is not subject to first-pass metabolism, and the other half via the stomach and intestine. The terminal elimination half-life is 7–8 hours, slightly longer than after IV injection. However, the major determinant of the duration of action is the redistribution of the drug into tissues, as after IV

Table 6.3 Main pharmacokinetic indices for OTFC, oral and IV fentanyl (using a dose of 15 µg/kg)

	C_{max} (ng/ml)	t_{max} (minutes)	$t_{1/2}$ (minutes)	Bioavailability %
IV	–	–	425 ± 102	–
OTFC	3.0 ± 1.0	22 ± 2.5	460 ± 313	52 ± 10
Oral	1.6 ± 0.6	101 ± 48.8	469 ± 123	32 ± 10

C_{max} = peak plasma concentration

t_{max} = time to peak plasma concentration

$t_{1/2}$ = elimination half-life

Source: Streisand *et al.* (1991)

administration. The rapid absorption and time to peak plasma concentrations are associated with an even more rapid onset of pain relief of 5–10 minutes (Sevarino *et al.* 1997), and the duration of effect is about two hours.

Clinical efficacy

The quick onset and short duration of analgesia produced by OTFC is an ideal profile for managing acute episodic pain in cancer patients. One of the most difficult types of pain to treat in this group of patients is pain on weight-bearing or movement. As discussed above, normal-release morphine has limitations in dealing with this sort of pain and there are other causes of 'breakthrough' pain which present similar difficulties. Several studies have been completed in cancer patients maintained on regular opioid analgesics who experience acute episodic pain and have demonstrated that OTFC is effective and well tolerated in this indication and is superior to normal-release morphine (Christie *et al.* 1998; Farrar *et al.* 1998; Portenoy *et al.* 1999). OTFC is not yet licensed in Europe but should be in the near future. It appears to be an important addition to the available opioids for the specific indication of 'break-through' pain.

Oxycodone

Oxycodone is a semi-synthetic congener of morphine, which has been on the market for 80 years but until recently was only available in formulations which effectively circumscribed its use. In the USA it has been prescribed in low-dose combination products with a non-opioid for oral administration, and in the UK only a rectal suppository and no oral formulations have been available. In some other countries parenteral oxycodone has had an important role as a post-operative analgesic: in Finland it has been the most commonly used post-operative opioid (Kalso *et al.* 1991). These variable availability and variable use have resulted in some confusion about its efficacy and potency, particularly in cancer pain management. Until now oxycodone has been viewed primarily as a step-2 opioid because it was first introduced in the USA in low-dose opioid/non-opioid combination products, and this is where such products have been positioned. In the UK, rectal oxycodone has had limited use as an alternative to morphine for patients unable to take oral medication. Oxycodone has been more widely used by mouth as a first-line step-3 opioid in other countries, particularly in Scandinavia, and it is now about to become widely available as a single agent in new oral formulations in many different countries. This development is likely to bring about substantial changes in the way it is used and in its role as an alternative to morphine.

Pharmacokinetics

The pharmacokinetics of oxycodone have only recently been described. It is well absorbed after oral administration and has a bioavailability of 60–87 per cent (Leow et al. 1992; Pöyhiä et al. 1992). It is metabolised in the liver to noroxycodone and oxymorphone and various glucuronide conjugates (Cone et al. 1984; Pöyhiä et al. 1993). A small proportion, 8–14 per cent, is excreted unchanged in the urine. Both major metabolites have some pharmacological activity and it has been proposed that oxymorphone contributes to the analgesic effects of oxycodone (Inturrisi 1990). However, this metabolite is produced in very small quantities; and a recent study provides additional evidence that it does not contribute to the pharmacological effects of oxycodone in humans. O-demethylation of oxycodone to oxymorphone is catalysed by the enzyme cytochrome P450 2D6 (CYP2D6), which can be blocked by quinidine. In a study in healthy subjects (Heiskanen et al. 1998), blocking the production of oxymorphone with quinidine had no effect on the psychomotor or subjective effects of oxycodone (analgesia was not evaluated). Current evidence suggests, therefore, that the metabolites of oxycodone do not contribute significantly to its pharmacological effects. The elimination half-life of oxycodone is 2–5 hours.

Pharmacology and clinical efficacy

Oxycodone has relatively weak affinity for the μ-receptor: approximately one-tenth to one-fortieth that of morphine (Chen et al. 1991). However, it may be that the analgesic effects of oxycodone are primarily mediated by κ-opioid receptors and this may be the basis for a slightly different spectrum of activity compared with morphine (Ross & Smith 1997). There has been considerable confusion about the relative analgesic potency of oxycodone and part of the explanation is that the relative potency of oxycodone appears to differ with different routes of administration (Pöyhiä et al. 1993). Early studies using single intramuscular doses in post-operative pain models found that the analgesic potency of oxycodone was two-thirds to three-quarters that of morphine (Beaver et al. 1978a, 1978b). However, a more recent study indicated that lower doses of intravenous oxycodone were required for post-operative pain relief compared with morphine (Kalso et al. 1991). The greater oral bioavailability of oxycodone compared with morphine may also contribute to its greater potency when administered by mouth with a relative potency of between 4:3 and 2:1 (Kalso & Vainio 1990; Bruera *et al.* 1998).

These different reported ratios have contributed to the confusion about where oxycodone fits in the analgesic ladder. It has been used mainly at step-2 but also at step-3. This illustrates a point highlighted in the revised edition of *Cancer Pain Relief* from the WHO (1996). The old terminology of 'weak' and 'strong' opioids referring to analgesics used at step-2 or step-3 is an arbitrary division of this group of drugs since there is no fundamental difference between them. Thus the new recommended terminology is 'opioids for mild-to-moderate pain' and 'opioids for moderate-to-severe pain'. Oxycodone clearly spans both step-2 and step-3 but this applies to other opioids of similar efficacy such as morphine.

The new modified-release formulation of oxycodone has been designed to produce a biphasic absorption process with an initial rapid component (Mandema *et al.* 1996), which seems to be associated with an onset of analgesia similar to that produced by normal-release oxycodone (Sunshine *et al.* 1996). The aim is to facilitate the use of this formulation in the dose titration phase, but there is insufficient clinical experience with this product to know whether this will produce real benefits in practice.

Thus oxycodone is an old drug in a new guise. It is an effective alternative to morphine, which offers the promise of being more similar to morphine than any other drug and with some potential advantages: particularly its greater oral bioavailability. More data and experience with the new oral formulations are required to see whether oxycodone is effective over as wide a dose range as morphine and whether there are any differences in its side-effect profile. If it proves to be morphine with a different label, it is likely to have a major impact.

Other opioid analgesics

The agonist-antagonist opioid analgesics are a heterogeneous group of drugs with moderate-to-strong analgesic activity comparable to that of the agonist opioids such as codeine and morphine, but with a limited effective dose range. The group includes drugs which act as an agonist or partial agonist at one receptor and as an antagonist at another (pentazocine, butorphanol, nalbuphine, dezocine) and drugs acting as a partial agonist at a single receptor (buprenorphine). Nalbuphine is not available for oral use and butorphanol was withdrawn from the market in the UK some years ago. Pentazocine has weak analgesic effects by mouth. Thus the place of this group of drugs in chronic cancer pain is limited (Hoskin & Hanks 1991). Buprenorphine may have a place in patients in whom the sublingual route is preferable because of swallowing difficulties, but the maximum dose that can be given at any one time is limited by the number of tablets that a patient can tolerate sublingually.

Dextromoramide and phenazocine are potent opioids (twice and five times as potent by mouth as morphine, respectively). However, there are no published RCTs of either drug and there is generally limited information about their pharmacokinetics and clinical efficacy. Dextromoramide has a very short duration of action and has been used for 'breakthrough' pain, but it does not have major advantages over morphine when used in this way. Phenazocine has been used as an alternative to morphine and can be given either orally or sublingually, but its use has declined with the introduction of hydromorphone.

Papaveretum is a combination of morphine with other opium alkaloids (predominantly noscapine with small amounts of codeine and papaverine). There is no evidence that it has any advantages over morphine alone. Dipipanone is a diphenylpropylamine structurally related to dextromoramide and methadone. It is only available in the UK in a combination tablet containing 10 mg of dipipanone and 30 mg of cyclizine, which limits its use.

In the last decade there has been interest in developing selective κ-agonists and more recently selective δ-agonists. The motivation is to produce powerful analgesics without the serious adverse effects associated with the standard drugs such as morphine. To some extent this has been rather misguided in that the particular adverse effects which worry pharmacologists (respiratory depression and tolerance and addiction) are not relevant problems when these drugs are used clinically to manage cancer pain. No selective κ-agonists have made it as far as the market but there are various δ-agonists in phase-II clinical trials at present. However, they are still some way from the clinic.

Conclusions

Morphine is the prototype opioid analgesic and remains the first choice step-3 opioid for chronic cancer pain management. Of the available alternatives, hydromorphone is the most useful and flexible and it may have a particular advantage in patients with renal impairment. Oxycodone promises much and may prove to be of great importance in the future but there remains relatively little experience with it in its new oral formulations. Transdermal fentanyl has a place in patients with stable opioid requirements or in patients who are having major problems with constipation, and oral transmucosal fentanyl citrate is an important addition for the management of acute episodic pain.

References

Ahmedzai S & Brooks D (1997). Transdermal fentanyl versus sustained-release oral morphine in cancer pain: preference, efficacy and quality of life. *Journal of Pain and Symptom Management* **13**, 254–61.

Babul N, Darke AC & Hagen N (1995). Hydromorphone metabolite accumulation in renal failure. *Journal of Pain and Symptom Management* **10**, 184–5.

Bartlett SE & Smith MT (1995). The apparent affinity of morphine-3-glucuronide for mu_1-opioid receptors results from morphine contamination: demonstration using HPLC and radioligand binding. *Life Sciences* **57**, 609–15.

Beaver WT, Wallenstein SL, Rogers A & Houde R (1978a). Analgesic studies of codeine and oxycodone in patients with cancer. I. Comparisons of oral with intramuscular codeine and of oral with intramuscular oxycodone. *Journal of Pharmacology and Experimental Therapeutics* **207**, 92–100.

Beaver WT, Wallenstein SL, Rogers A & Houde R (1978b). Analgesic studies of codeine and oxycodone in patients with cancer. II. Comparisons of intramuscular oxycodone with intramuscular morphine. *Journal of Pharmacology and Experimental Therapeutics* **207**, 101–8.

Bruera E, Sloan P, Mount B *et al.* (1996). A randomized, double-blind, double-dummy, crossover trial comparing the safety and efficacy of oral sustained-release hydromorphone with immediate-release hydromorphone in patients with cancer pain. Canadian Palliative Care Clinical Trials Group. *Journal of Clinical Oncology* **14**, 1713–17.

Bruera E, Belzile, Pituskin E *et al.* (1998). Randomized, double-blind, cross-over trial comparing safety and efficacy of oral controlled-release oxycodone with controlled-release morphine in patients with cancer pain. *Journal of Clinical Oncology* **16**, 3222–9.

Chaplan SR, Duncan SR, Brodsky JB & Brose WG (1992). Morphine and hydromorphone epidural analgesia. *Anesthesiology* **77**, 1090–4.

Chen ZR, Irvine RJ, Somogyi AA & Bochner F (1991). Mu receptor binding of some commonly used opioids and their metabolites. *Life Sciences* **48**, 2165–71.

Christie JM, Simmonds M, Patt R *et al.* (1998). Dose-titration, multicenter study of oral transmucosal fentanyl citrate for the treatment of breakthrough pain in cancer patients using transdermal fentanyl for persistent pain. *Journal of Clinical Oncology* **16**, 3238–45.

Cone EJ, Phelps BA & Gorodetzky CW (1977). Urinary excretion of hydromorphone and metabolites in humans, rats, dogs, guinea pigs, and rabbits. *Journal of Pharmaceutical Sciences* **66**, 1709–13.

Cone EJ, Darwin WD, Buchwald WF *et al.* (1984). Comparative metabolism and excretion of oxycodone in man and laboratory animals. *Federal Proceedings* **43**, 655.

de Stoutz ND, Bruera E & Suarez-Almazor M (1995). Opioid rotation for toxicity reduction in terminal cancer patients. *Journal of Pain and Symptom Management* **10**, 378–84.

Donner B, Zenz M, Tryba M & Strumpf M (1996). Direct conversion from oral morphine to transdermal fentanyl: a multicenter study in patients with cancer pain. *Pain* **64**, 527–34.

Donner B, Zenz M, Strumpf M & Raber M (1998). Long-term treatment of cancer pain with transdermal fentanyl. *Journal of Pain and Symptom Management* **15**, 168–75.

Ettinger DS, Vitale PJ & Trump DL (1979). Important clinical pharmacologic considerations in the use of methadone in cancer patients. *Cancer Treatment Reports* **63**, 457–9.

Fainsinger R, Schoeller T & Bruera E (1993). Methadone in the management of cancer pain: a review. *Pain* **52**, 137–47.

Fainsinger R & Toro R (1998). Opioids, confusion and opioid rotation. *Palliative Medicine* **12**, 463–4.

Farrar JT, Cleary J, Rauck, Busch M & Nordbrock E (1998). Oral transmucosal fentanyl citrate: randomised, double-blinded, placebo-controlled trial for treatment of breakthrough pain in cancer patients. *Journal of the National Cancer Institute* **90**, 611–16.

Faura CC, Collins SL, Moore RA & McQuay HJ (1998). Systematic review of factors affecting the ratios of morphine and its major metabolites. *Pain* **74**, 43–53.

Fine PG (1997). Fentanyl in the treatment of cancer pain. *Seminars in Oncology* **24**, (Suppl.16), S20–7.

Glare PA & Walsh D (1991). Clinical pharmacokinetics of morphine. *Therapeutic Drug Monitoring* **13**, 1–23.

Goisis A, Gorini M, Ratti R & Luliri P (1989). Application of a WHO protocol on medical therapy for oncologic pain in an internal medicine hospital. *Tumori* **75**, 470–2.

Gorman A, Elliott K & Inturrisi CE (1997). The d- and l- isomers of methadone bind to the non-competitive site on the N-methyl-D-aspartate (NMDA) receptor in rat forebrain and spinal cord. *Neurosciences Letter* **223**, 5–8.

Grochow L, Sheidler V, Grossman S *et al.* (1989). Does intravenous methadone provide longer lasting analgesia than intravenous morphine? A randomised double blind study. *Pain* **38**, 151–7.

Grond S, Zech D, Lehmann KA *et al.* (1997). Transdermal fentanyl in the long-term treatment of cancer pain: a prospective study of 50 patients with advanced cancer of the gastrointestinal tract or the head and neck region. *Pain* **69**, 191–8.

Haazen L, Noorduin H, Megens A *et al.* (1999). The constipation-inducing potential of morphine and transdermal fentanyl. *European Journal of Pain* **3**(Suppl.A), 9–15.

Hanks GW (1990). Controlled-release morphine tablets in chronic cancer pain: a review of controlled clinical trials. In *Advances in pain research and therapy* vol. 12 (ed. C Benedetti, CR Chapman & G Giron), pp.269–74. Raven Press, New York , USA.

Hanks GW, Hoskin PJ, Aherne GW, Turner P & Poulain P (1987). Explanation for the potency of repeated oral doses of morphine? *Lancet* **2**, 723–4.

Hanks GW & Fallon MT (1995). Transdermal fentanyl in cancer pain: conversion from oral morphine. *Journal of Pain and Symptom Management* **10**, 87.

Hanks GW, De Conno F, Ripamonti C *et al.* (1996). Morphine in cancer pain: modes of administration. *BMJ* **312**, 823–6.

Hanks GW & Forbes K (1997). Opioid responsiveness. *Acta Anaesthesiologica Scandinavica* **41**, 154–8.

Hawley P, Forbes K & Hanks GW (1998). Opioids, confusion and opioid rotation. *Palliative Medicine* **12**, 63–4.

Hays H, Hagen N, Thirlwell M *et al.* (1994). Comparative clinical efficacy and safety of immediate release and controlled release hydromorphone for chronic severe cancer pain. *Cancer* **74**, 1808–16.

Heiskanen T, Olkkola KT & Kalso E (1998). Effects of blocking CYP 2D6 on the pharmacokinetics and pharmacodynamics of oxycodone. *Clinical Pharmacology and Therapeutics* **64**, 603–11.

Hess R, Steibler G & Herz A (1972). Pharmacokinetics of fentanyl in man and the rabbit. *European Journal of Clinical Pharmacology* **4**, 135–41.

Hoskin PJ, Hanks GW, Aherne GW, Chapman D, Littleton P & Filshie J (1989). The bioavailability and pharmacokinetics of morphine after intravenous, oral and buccal administration in healthy volunteers. *British Journal of Clinical Pharmacology* **27**, 499–505.

Hoskin PJ & Hanks GW (1990). Morphine: pharmacokinetics and clinical practice. *British Journal of Cancer* **62**, 705–7.

Hoskin PJ & Hanks GW (1991). Opioid agonist-antagonist drugs in acute and chronic pain states. *Drugs* **41**, 326–44.

Houde RW (1986). Clinical analgesic studies of hydromorphone. In *Advances in pain research and therapy* vol. 8 (ed. KM Foley & CE Inturrisi), pp.129–35. Raven Press, New York, USA.

Inturrisi CE (1990). Effects of other drugs and pathologic states on opioid disposition and response. In *Advances in pain research and therapy* vol. 12 (ed. C Benedetti, CR Chapman & G Giron), pp.171–80. Raven Press, New York, USA.

Inturrisi CE & Verebely K (1972). Disposition of methadone in man after a single oral dose. *Clinical Pharmacology and Therapeutics* **13**, 923–30.

Inturrisi C, Portenoy R, Stillman M *et al.* (1988). Hydromorphone bioavailability and pharmacokinetic-pharmacodynamic (PK-PD) relationships (abst. POII-2). *Clinical Pharmacology and Therapeutics* **43**, 162.

Jadad AR & Browman GP (1995). The WHO analgesic ladder for cancer pain management. *Journal of the American Medical Association* **274**, 1870–3.

Kalso E & Vainio A (1990). Morphine and oxycodone hydrochloride in the management of cancer pain. *Clinical Pharmacology and Therapeutics* **47**, 639–46.

Kalso E, Pöyhiä R, Onnela P, Linko K, Tigerstedt I & Tammisto T (1991). Intravenous morphine and oxycodone for pain after abdominal surgery. *Acta Anaesthesiologica Scandinavica* **35**, 642–6.

Lehmann KA & Zech D (1992). Transdermal fentanyl: clinical pharmacology. *Journal of Pain and Symptom Management* **7**(Suppl.), S8–16.

Leow KP, Smith MT, Williams B & Cramond T (1992). Single-dose and steady-state pharmacokinetics and pharmacodynamics of oxycodone in patients with cancer. *Clinical Pharmacology and Therapeutics* **52**, 487–95.

Mandema JW, Kaiko RF, Oshlack B, Reder RF & Stanski DR (1996). Characterization and validation of a pharmacokinetic model for controlled-release oxycodone. *British Journal of Clinical Pharmacology* **42**, 747–56.

Mather LE (1983). Clinical pharmacokinetics of fentanyl and its newer derivatives. *Clinical Pharmacokinetics* **8**, 422–46.

McClain DA & Hug CC (1980). Intravenous fentanyl kinetics. *Clinical Pharmacology and Therapeutics* **28**, 106–14.

McDonald CJ & Miller AJ (1997). A comparative potency study of a controlled release tablet formulation of hydromorphone and controlled release morphine in patients with cancer pain. European Association for Palliative Care 5th Congress, London. Book of Abstracts S37.

Megens A, Artois K, Vermeire J *et al.* (1998). Comparison of the analgesic and intestinal effects of fentanyl and morphine in rats. *Journal of Pain and Symptom Management* **15**, 253–7.

Osborne R, Joel S & Slevin M (1986). Morphine intoxication in renal failure: the role of morphine-6-glucuronide. *British Medical Journal* **292**, 1548–9.

Pohland A, Boaz HE & Sullivan HR (1971). Synthesis and identification of metabolites resulting from the biotransformation of d,l-methadone in man and in the rat. *Journal of Medicinal Chemistry* **14**, 194–7.

Portenoy RK, Southam MA, Gupta SK *et al.* (1993). Transdermal fentanyl for cancer pain. Repeated dose pharmacokinetics. *Anesthesiology* **78**, 36–43.

Portenoy RK, Payne R, Coluzzi P *et al.* (1999). Oral transmucosal fentanyl citrate (OTFC) for the treatment of breakthrough pain in cancer patients: a controlled dose titration study. *Pain* **79**, 303–12.

Pöyhiä R, Seppälä T, Olkkola KT & Kalso E (1992). The pharmacokinetics and metabolism of oxycodone after intramuscular and oral administration to healthy subjects. *British Journal of Clinical Pharmacology* **33**, 617–21.

Pöyhiä R, Vainio A & Kalso E (1993). A review of oxycodone's clinical pharmacokinetics and pharmacodynamics. *Journal of Pain and Symptom Management* **8**, 63–7.

Ripamonti C, Groff L, Brunelli C *et al.* (1998). Switching from morphine to oral methadone in treating cancer pain: what is the equianalgesic dose ratio? *Journal of Clinical Oncology* **16**, 3216–21.

Rosow CE, Moss J, Philbin DM *et al.* (1982). Histamine release during morphine and fentanyl anesthesia. *Anesthesiology* **56**, 93–6.

Ross FB & Smith MT (1997). The intrinsic antinociceptive effects of oxycodone appear to be κ-opioid receptor mediated. *Pain* **73**, 151–7.

Sevarino FB, Ginsberg B, Lichtor JL *et al.* (1997). Oral transmucosal fentanyl citrate (OTFC) compared with IV morphine for acute pain in patients following abdominal surgery. *Anesthesia and Analgesia* **84**, S330.

Shimomura K, Kamata O, Ueki S *et al.* (1971). Analgesic effect of morphine glucuronides. *Tohuku Journal of Experimental Medicine* **105**, 45–52.

Siguan SS, Damole AA & Mejarito AG (1992). Results of cancer pain treatment at Southern Islands Medical Centre, Cebu, Philippines. *Philippine Journal of Surgical Specialties* **47**, 173–6.

Sloan PA, Moulin DE & Hays H (1998). A clinical evaluation of transdermal therapeutic system fentanyl for the treatment of cancer pain. *Journal of Pain and Symptom Management* **16**, 102–11.

Storey P (1995). More on the conversion of transdermal fentanyl to morphine. *Journal of Pain and Symptom Management* **10**, 581.

Streisand JB, Varvel JR, Stanski DR *et al.* (1991). Absorption and bioavailability of oral transmucosal fentanyl citrate. *Anesthesiology* **75**, 223–9.

Sunshine A, Olson NZ, Colon A *et al.* (1996). Analgesic efficacy of controlled-release oxycodone in postoperative pain. *Journal of Clinical Pharmacology* **36**, 595–603

Takeda F (1990). Japan's WHO cancer pain relief program. In *Advances in pain research and therapy* vol. 16 (ed. KM Foley, JJ Bonica, V Ventafridda & MV Callaway), pp.475–483. Raven Press, New York, USA.

Uhl GR, Sora I & Wang Z (1999). The mu opiate receptor as a candidate gene for pain: polymorphisms, variations in expression, nociception, and opiate responses. *Proceedings of the National Academy of Sciences of the USA* **96**, 7752–5.

Vallner JJ, Stewart JT, Kotzan JA *et al.* (1981). Pharmacokinetics and bioavailability of hydromorphone following intravenous and oral administration to human subjects. *Journal of Clinical Pharmacology* **21**, 152–6.

Varvel JR, Shafer SL, Hwang SS *et al.* (1989). Absorption characteristics of transdermally administered fentanyl. *Anesthesiology* **70**, 928–34.

Ventafridda V, Ripamonti C, Bianchi M *et al.* (1986). A randomised study on oral administration of morphine and methadone in the treatment of cancer pain. *Journal of Pain and Symptom Management* **1**, 203–8.

Ventafridda V, Tamburini M, Caraceni A, De Conno F & Naldi F (1987). A validation study of the WHO method for cancer pain relief. *Cancer* **59**, 850–6.

Ventafridda V, Caraceni A & Gamba A (1990). Field-testing of the WHO guidelines for cancer pain relief. In *Advances in pain research and therapy* vol. 16 (ed. KM Foley, JJ Bonica, V Ventafridda & MV Callaway), pp.451–64. Raven Press, New York, USA.

Verebely K, Volavka J, Mule S & Resnick R (1975). Methadone in man: pharmacokinetic and excretion studies in acute and chronic treatment. *Clinical Pharmacology and Therapeutics* **18**, 180–90.

Walker VA, Hoskin PJ, Hanks GW & White ID (1988). Evaluation of WHO analgesic guidelines for cancer pain in a hospital-based palliative care unit. *Journal of Pain and Symptom Management* **3**, 145–9.

Wenk R, Diaz C, Echeverria M *et al.* (1991). Argentina's WHO cancer pain relief program: a patient care model. *Journal of Pain and Symptom Management* **6**, 40–3.

World Health Organization (1996). *Cancer pain relief* 2nd edition. WHO, Geneva.

Yeadon M & Kitchen I (1988). Comparative binding of μ and δ selective ligands in whole brain and pons/medulla homogenates from rat: affinity profiles of fentanyl derivatives. *Neuropharmacology* **27**, 345–8.

Yeh SY, Gorodetsky CW & Krebs HA (1977). Isolation and identification of morphine 3- and 6-glucuronides, morphine 3,6-diglucuronide, morphine 3-ethereal sulphate, normorphine, and normorphine 6-glucuronide as morphine metabolites in humans. *Journal of Pharmaceutical Sciences* **66**, 1288–93.

Yeo W, Lam KK, Chan ATC, Leung TWT, Nip SYW & Johnson PJ (1997). Transdermal fentanyl for severe cancer-related pain. *Palliative Medicine* **11**, 233–9.

Zech DFJ, Grond S, Lynch J, Hertel D & Lehmann KA (1995). Validation of World Health Organization guidelines for cancer pain relief: a 10-year prospective study. *Pain* **63**, 65–76.

Zenz M, Donner B & Strumpf M (1994). Withdrawal symptoms during therapy with transdermal fentanyl (Fentanyl TTS)? *Journal of Pain and Symptom Management* **9**, 54–5.

Chapter 7

Recent progress in the use of non-steroidal analgesia: the place of old and new NSAIDs

Anthony Byrne

Introduction

Non-steroidal anti-inflammatory drugs (NSAIDs) represent a diverse group of therapeutic agents which have gained universal acceptance in the treatment of inflammatory and painful conditions. They fall into several chemical groups and are marketed in multiple formulations, being responsible for over 20 million prescriptions a year in the UK (5 per cent of total NHS prescriptions) and accounting for a world market in excess of $6 billion per year (Garner 1992).

Acetylsalicylic acid is the prototypical commercialised NSAID. It was synthesised in 1899 by Felix Hofferman of the Bayer Corporation and named 'aspirin' by its chief pharmacologist Herman Dreser (1899). Plant extracts containing salicylic acid had been used for centuries for the treatment of pain and fever, so that aspirin's commercial and clinical success was unsurprising. It was not until much later, however, that a clear understanding of its pharmacodynamics emerged. A study published by Vane (1971) demonstrated that aspirin and other NSAIDs act by blocking prostaglandin synthesis through inhibition of the enzyme prostaglandin G/H synthase, colloquially known as cyclooxygenase (Cox). This biochemical activity was proposed to account not only for the therapeutic effects of these drugs but also their adverse-effect profile, which had clearly emerged in the years following their introduction (Coles *et al.* 1983). Cox was ascribed important housekeeping functions as a constitutively expressed enzyme, including gastric mucosal protection and vascular homeostasis, its interruption therefore having significant pathophysiological implications.

The complex relationship between drug and enzyme became even more intriguing with the discovery in 1991 of a second isoform, designated Cox-2 (Xie *et al.* 1991). Evidence quickly accumulated that this enzyme was induced by mitogenic and inflammatory stimuli (Herschman 1996) rather than being constitutively expressed raising the possibility of differential Cox inhibition and minimisation of the side-effects associated with blockade of Cox-1. Such promise has led to the development of a new generation of NSAIDs aimed at specific Cox-2 inhibition with potentially enormous clinical and economic implications (Vane 1994; Service 1996). This chapter will review the biological activity of 'old' and 'new' NSAIDs, evidence of their clinical efficacy and their respective roles in the treatment of cancer pain.

Prostaglandin G/H synthase (cyclooxygenase) structure and activity

The rate-limiting step in the formation of eicosanoids is the release of arachidonic acid from membrane phospholipids. This is achieved through phospholipase A_2 (Figure 7.1), representing a family of hydrolysing enzymes which may be activated by various external signals, including the inflammatory mediators bradykinin, norepinephrine and thrombin (Herschman 1998). The release of precursor, which is inhibited by corticosteroids, has traditionally been recognised as the route for involvement of prostaglandins in inflammatory and pain processes, providing adequate substrate for increased Cox activity.

Cox catalyses the first committed step in the production of prostaglandins (Figure 7.1). This haem-containing enzyme exhibits two distinct activities: the eponymous Cox activity which extracts a hydrogen from arachidonic acid (AA) to form the hydroperoxide PGG_2, and a peroxidase activity which reduces PGG_2 to the endoperoxide PGH_2. These events occur at two distinct but apparently interacting sites, located as a globular catalytic domain in the main body of the enzyme.

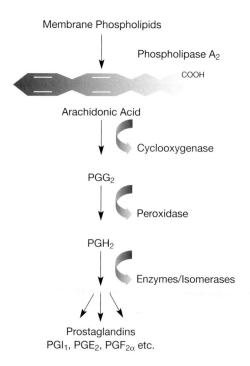

Membrane Phospholipids

Phospholipase A_2

COOH

Arachidonic Acid

Cyclooxygenase

PGG_2

Peroxidase

PGH_2

Enzymes/Isomerases

Prostaglandins
PGI_1, PGE_2, $PGF_{2\alpha}$ etc.

Figure 7.1 Pathway of prostaglandin production

X-ray crystallographic studies of Cox-1 have provided great insight into the structure/function relationships of the enzyme (Picot *et al.* 1994). They show that the Cox site consists of a long, hydrophobic channel with a tyosine residue (Tyr385) at its apex (Figure 7.2a), nestled near the edge of the haem plane. The channel also contains a serine residue close by at position 530 and an arginine lower down at position 120. The positioning of the enzyme allows AA access to the hydrophobic channel from the interior of the phospholipid bilayer. The arginine represents a rare polar residue in this hydrophobic corridor, a suitable candidate to bind the carbohydrate group of AA, allowing it to dock and curve the C-13 hydrogen into the proposed catalytic domain higher up.

Initiation of Cox activity requires hydroperoxide, thought to derive from the peroxidase catalytic cycle. It is suggested that this produces a tyrosyl radical capable of extracting the hydrogen atom from AA, with subsequent production of the endoperoxide intermediates and prostaglandin end products. Any attempt to interfere with this process would therefore logically involve prohibition of AA access to the channel, prevention of tyrosyl radical production or dissociation of Cox and peroxidase activity. It is the first of these which appears to form the mechanism of action of conventional NSAIDs.

Mechanism of action of NSAIDs

NSAIDs inhibit prostaglandin synthesis by blocking the Cox channel about halfway down (Lanzo *et al.* 1998), preventing AA access to the critical apical domain (Figure 7.2b). Given the diverse chemical structure of NSAIDs, it is not surprising that there

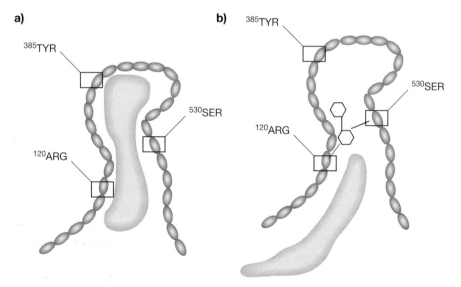

Figure 7.2 Cartoon of structure of the active site of cyclooxygenase, with (a) access of AA along the hydrophobic channel, and (b) action of NSAIDs in prohibiting access

are several types of such inhibition. Aspirin produces a rapid, irreversible inhibition of Cox-1 by acetylation of a serine residue at position 530. This covalent modification produces a bulky sidegroup preventing AA movement towards tyrosine 385 (Loll *et al.* 1995). Drugs such as indomethicin, diclofenac and flurbiprofen, on the other hand, produce a time-dependent irreversible inhibition through salt bridge formation between a carboxylic acid group and Arg120 of the enzyme channel (Mancini *et al.* 1995). This both physically hinders access to the upper channel and also competitively inhibits anchorage of AA to Arg120 via its own carboxylate group. Ibuprofen and mefanamic acid cause rapid, reversible inhibition via competition with AA without forming a product with, or structural change in, the enzyme. Potency of individual NSAIDs varies considerably with inhibitory concentration (IC50) values (μM) for Cox-1 *ex vivo,* ranging from 3.2 for aspirin to 0.037 for diclofenac (Kawai *et al.*1998).

Mechanisms of NSAID analgesic activity

Traditionally, non-steroidal anti-inflammatories have been ascribed a peripheral mechanism of action in their role as analgesics and modulators of inflammation. However, abundant evidence now exists to also support centrally mediated effects. Inflammatory processes are often associated with pain and hyperalgesia and are subserved by a complex interaction in the periphery between immune cells and neural elements (Dray 1995). This environment includes cytokine, histamine and serotonin release by immune cells and highly reactive neuropeptides such as calcitonon gene-related peptide and substance P, resulting in direct stimulation or sensitisation of nociceptors. Prostaglandins released by neurons and polymorphs represent a potent link in the co-ordination of this response, and inhibition of PGE_2 and PGI_2 by NSAIDs would logically dampen this significantly (Cashman 1996).

Animal and human studies suggest a central mechanism of analgesic activity to augment the peripheral effect of NSAIDs. Studies in rats have shown that NSAIDs can block the hyperalgesia mediated by spinal glutamate and substance P, implying a role for prostaglandins in the facilitated state of spinal processing associated with protracted C fibre barrage (Malmberg *et al.* 1992). Furthermore, thalamic-evoked responses to electrical stimulation of nociceptive afferents are depressed by central activity of several NSAIDs (Carlsson *et al.* 1988; Jurna *et al.* 1992), intrathecal lysine acetylsalicylate has been reported to abolish pain in man (Devoghel 1983), and centrally applied acetylsalicylic acid inhibits meningeal nociception in rats (Ellrich *et al.* 1999).

Opioidergic and serotonergic mechanisms have additionally been proposed for central NSAID activity. Inhibition of NSAID antinociception by naloxone has been equated with evidence of involvement with opioid systems, but this may represent indirect rather than direct interaction (Bjorkman 1995). Diclofenac has also been shown to activate descending serotonin pathways to elicit analgesia, possibly via a 5-HT_2 receptor mechanism (McCormack 1994).

Clinical efficacy of NSAIDs for cancer pain

NSAIDs are universally accepted as part of the treatment of cancer-related pain, occupying a central role in WHO guidelines on cancer pain relief (World Health Organization 1992). Despite their long history of use for non-malignant pain, reports of analgesic effect in oncological diseases were sparse until Stoll (1973) described an effect of indomethicin in breast cancer patients with bony metastases. Since then a number of studies have sought to examine the efficacy of NSAIDs versus other analgesics or placebo in a range of malignant conditions. Given the widespread acceptance of NSAIDs for pain control based on the assumptions of clinical experience, large-scale trials have not taken place. However, Eisenburg *et al.* (1994) have attempted to collate the available data by meta-analysis of published randomised controlled trials. They analysed 25 randomised, double-blind controlled studies published between 1974 and 1990. They included single- and multiple-dose studies and parallel and crossover designs. Twenty-one were single-centre. The analysis gave data on 1,545 patients, although a specific cancer diagnosis was only described for one third of these. Only single-dose studies were combinable for analgesic efficacy analysis. They suggested a statistically significant difference in pain control for NSAIDs over placebo – resulting in approximately twice as much analgesia. Six studies made comparison with 'weak' opioids and three with 5–10 mg of intramuscular morphine. There was no significant difference in efficacy between NSAIDs and either alternative. There were very limited data on dose-response relationships, but data on the use of recommended versus supramaximal doses of three drugs indicated a ceiling effect for analgesia. Overall, studies did not report outcome in relation to cancer type, but pain was related to bone metastases in seven series. Only two were evaluable but not combinable (single versus multiple dose), and suggested efficacy similar to non-bone malignant pain. Side-effects occurred less frequently than with 'weak' or 'strong' opioids in single-dose studies, but there appeared to be a dose-related effect.

This was a thorough and detailed review but was hampered by a number of issues. Only published trials were used, introducing an inevitable bias. Although weighting was given to larger trials, quality of trials was not graded and therefore low and high quality series were analysed together. Analysis of *statistical* significance needs also to be interpreted with caution as many reports did not provide broad statistical information and rough approximations (e.g. of standard deviations) were therefore made. Nonetheless important evidence of *clinically* significant improvements was shown, with a peak pain relief incidence of 60 per cent in patients who reported baseline pain as moderate or severe.

Adverse effects associated with NSAIDs

Chronic use of NSAIDs is associated with a significant incidence of gastrointestinal (GI) and renal toxicity. Estimated annual US costs associated with NSAID toxicity are in the region of $1.3 billion (McGoldrick *et al.* 1997).

Gastroenteropathy is the most commonly described adverse effect, first reported for acetylsalicyclic acid by Douthwaite *et al.* (1938). The ability of an NSAID to produce gastric damage correlates with its ability to suppress gastric prostaglandin synthesis (Lanza 1989). Several factors may explain this. Prostaglandins mediate mucus and bicarbonate secretion, mucosal immunocyte activity and blood flow. Loss of prostaglandin synthesis may therefore lead to impairment of mucosal defence against luminal irritants. It is unclear, however, why Cox-1 knockout mice do not develop spontaneous gastric ulceration (Langenbach *et al.* 1995) if this is the main mechanism, or why the majority of patients taking NSAIDs do not develop gastroenteropathy despite profound gastric prostaglandin suppression. Other factors which may play a role include upregulation of intercellular adhesion molecule-1 (ICAM-1) in the gastric microcirculation and CD11/CD8 in circulating neutrophils and lowering of pH in the mucosal environment by these drugs (Wallace 1997).

Several studies have examined the likelihood of upper GI events in patients taking NSAIDs (Langman *et al.* 1994; Garcia Rodriguez *et al.* 1994; Møller Hansen *et al.* 1996) and suggest an excess risk of GI bleeding for NSAID users of 3.0–5.0 over non-users. Both Langman and Garcia Rodriguez produced large case control studies to assess the risk for individual drugs. Despite important differences in design (Langman identified 1,144 patients aged over 60 presenting to hospital with GI bleeding; Garcia Rodriguez used computerised GP records to identify 1,457 cases of GI bleeding or perforation with no age restriction), the results were very similar (Table 7.1).

Interestingly, Langman found no association with prior history of peptic ulcer disease. Although Garcia Rodriguez did, this appeared to be largely secondary to the spontaneously increased risk of this group whether taking NSAIDs or not. An association in the latter study of increased risk with increasing age is supported by other studies (Gabriel *et al.* 1991; Møller Hansen *et al.* 1996), although not by Langman, as is an approximately twofold increase in NSAID users taking concomitant corticosteroids over NSAID users alone (Møller Hansen *et al.* 1996). Although Langman saw an increased incidence of adverse events in those starting NSAID therapy in the previous month, others suggest the risk is constant over time (Silverstein *et al.* 1995; MacDonald *et al.* 1997).

Table 7.1

	Relative Risk	
	Garcia Rodriguez	*Langman*
Overall	4.7	4.5
Ibuprofen	2.9	2.0
Diclofenac	3.9	4.2
Naproxen	3.1	9.1

The effects of NSAIDs on renal function are less clearly defined. Prostaglandins have little role in renal homeostasis under euvolaemic conditions, but become critical in the setting of systemic or intrarenal circulatory disturbance. It is under such conditions that NSAIDs are likely to exacerbate the antidiuretic, antinatriuretic and vasoconstrictive effects of circulating angiotensin, vasopressin and catecholamines (Palmer 1995). NSAIDs may also exacerbate pre-existing renal dysfunction and age-related progressive decline in renal function. In a study of 1,908 patients treated with ibuprofen, the two most important predictors of decreased renal function were age over 65 and pre-existing renal failure (Murray *et al.* 1990). Whether most NSAIDs cause the sort of 'analgesic nephropathy' associated previously with phenacetin use remains unclear (Palmer 1995).

Avoidance of untoward effects of NSAIDs in the GI tract and kidneys may therefore depend on identification of individuals at high risk and the choice of specific NSAIDs at the lowest effective dose for the shortest possible period. Other approaches at limiting GI toxicity have until recently concentrated on concomitant suppression of acid secretion or administration of prostaglandin analogues. A meta-analysis of H_2-blockers and misoprostol in the prevention of gastric and duodenal lesions showed a significant benefit for misoprostol following short- and long-term treatment in reducing gastric lesions and for long-term treatment in reducing duodenal ulcers. No consistent benefit was seen for H_2-blockers (Koch *et al.* 1996). Although thorough and detailed, assessment of individual trial quality was limited and inclusion of lower-quality trials in the analysis may therefore overestimate treatment effectiveness. A Cochrane collaborative review group is currently reviewing the efficacy of H_2-blockers, proton pump inhibitors and prostaglandin analogues in preventing chronic NSAID-induced upper GI toxicity (Rostom 1999).

Cox-2 discovery – therapeutic implications

The discovery in 1991 of a second isoform of cyclooxygenase, Cox-2, which appeared to be induced by pro-inflammatory stimuli in a wide variety of tissues (Herschman 1996), heralded the intriguing possibility of differential inhibition of the enzyme. This could potentially provide anti-inflammatory and analgesic benefits without the side-effects traditionally associated with loss of Cox-1 activity. Both enzymes have approximately 60 per cent aminoacid sequence identity, share the same cyclooxygenase and peroxidase activities, have similar kinetics and share similar intracellular locations. They can, however, be selectively inhibited by certain compounds, and the elucidation of the X-ray crystal structure of human Cox-2 has allowed insight into possible mechanisms (Luong *et al.* 1996). This shows that overall structure is similar, and that Arg120 is conserved in Cox-2. However, the latter enzyme has an important amino acid difference at position 523: a valine which is smaller than the isoleucine 523 of Cox-1. The smaller residue allows access to a side pocket, which appears critical to selective inhibition (Figure 7.3). Drugs with bulky methyl, sulphone or sulphonamide can gain access to the Cox-2 channel because of this side pocket, but are too large to remain in the Cox-1 channel. Several selective inhibitors appear to produce short-lived reversible inhibition of Cox-1 and time-dependent irreversible inhibition of Cox-2 (Copeland *et al.* 1994).

Unsurprisingly, there has been enormous interest in development of Cox-2 inhibitors and several 'old' NSAIDs have been ascribed such selectivity. Tests of differential inhibition utilise various cell, pure enzyme or *ex vivo* whole blood assays.

Controversy over accuracy and applicability to *in vivo* conditions continue and estimates of selectivity may vary tenfold. In broad terms, drugs such as indomethicin and naproxen appear to have little selectivity for Cox-2, diclofenac is roughly equipotent for both isoforms (Kawai *et al.* 1998), while meloxicam is suggested to have some Cox-2 selectivity (Noble *et al.* 1996) and is therefore referred to as a preferential inhibitor of Cox-2. Cell-based screening assays and structure-aided drug development have led to a new generation of inhibitors which are at least 100 times as potent in inhibiting Cox-2 as Cox-1. One of these, SC58635 or celecoxib, has now been licensed in the USA for rheumatoid arthritis and osteoarthritis, with others likely to follow soon.

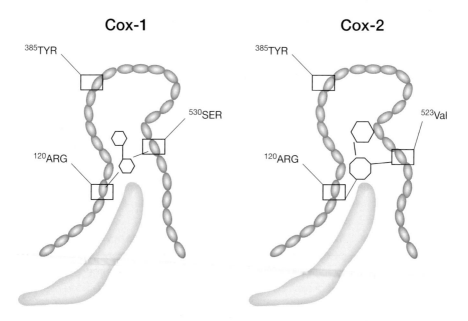

Figure 7.3 Cartoon of the hydrophobic channels of Cox-1 and Cox-2, highlighting the impact of valine substitution at position 523

Analgesic efficacy of Cox-2 inhibitors

Studies of analgesic efficacy for Cox-2 inhibitors have taken place in non-malignant conditions. A selection of such trials is shown in Table 7.2. As can be seen, comparison has tended to be with older NSAIDs from the more damaging end of the spectrum, such as piroxicam and naproxen at high doses. Study periods have tended to be relatively short and GI toxicity mainly based on symptoms rather than endoscopic findings. Meloxicam has been suggested to cause fewer adverse GI events than piroxicam (10.3 versus 15.4 per cent) in patients with osteoarthritis (Dequeker *et al.* 1998), while meloxicam and diclofenac had similar GI event rates (26.6 versus 27.7 per cent) in a similar patient group (Hosie *et al.* 1998). Although non-significant statistically, diclofenac was slightly more effective in reducing overall pain and pain on movement.

Experience with the Cox-2 specific inhibitors celecoxib and rofecoxib in phase III short-term studies of osteoarthritis suggests similar efficacy to naproxen (Hubbard 1998) and diclofenac (Cannon *et al.* 1998), respectively (see Table 7.2), for selected parameters such as patients' global assessment of pain and disease response. Long-term data on GI tolerability are awaited, but short-term studies suggest event rates similar to placebo (Hawkey 1999).

Cox-2 inhibition: potential risks for safety and efficacy

While highly selective Cox-2 inhibitors have great theoretical potential, several aspects of their behaviour in experimental studies and of the inflammatory/pain process, raise important issues of safety and efficacy. Many of the early clinical studies of gastric-sparing effects involved healthy volunteers, who are not reflective of the population, including the cancer population, likely to be prescribed these agents. There is emerging evidence from animal models, however, that Cox-2 may play an important protective role where GI mucosal damage already exists. It has been shown to be upregulated in rat models of gastric ulceration (Takahashi *et al.* 1998), ischaemic gastric damage (Mariolo *et al.* 1998) and models of experimental colitis (Reuter *et al.* 1996). Use of Cox-2 inhibitors in these settings has led to worsening of lesions and in the case of intestinal colitis, perforation and death of the animals.

Table 7.2

	Reference
Meloxicam 7.5 mg vs Piroxicam 20 mg	Dequeker *et al.* (1998)
Meloxicam 7.5 mg vs Diclofenac SR 100 mg	Hosie *et al.* (1996)
Celecoxib 200 mg vs Naproxen 1,000 mg	Hubbard *et al.* (1998)
Rofecoxib 12.5 mg vs Diclofenac 150 mg	Cannon *et al.* (1998)

Cox-2 is also constitutively expressed in the rat kidney and is upregulated under conditions of salt and water restriction (Harris RC *et al.* 1994), suggesting a role in modulation of renin activity in these conditions. Cox-2 knockout mice also display significant renal dysfunction and die before eight weeks of age due to poor renal maturation (Moreham *et al.* 1995). Such data suggest the need for clear information in varied patient groups before the long-term safety of these drugs can be assessed.

Analgesic efficacy of Cox-2 inhibitors also depends on a lack of involvement of Cox-1 in the inflammatory and pain processes. In experimental studies this may well depend on the model used. Also the doses of some Cox-2 inhibitors needed to exact an anti-inflammatory and analgesic effect in rat paw oedema assays have been shown to be in the range which also inhibits Cox-1. The degree of inflammation in Cox-2-deficient mice was comparable to wildtype littermates, confirming a role for Cox-1 (Wallace *et al.* 1998). A study of human bursitis suggests a similarly important role for Cox-1 in this inflammatory process (Gretzer *et al.* 1998).

Conclusion

NSAIDs have gained universal acceptance as analgesics in the treatment of cancer pain. Structural studies of the cyclooxygenase isoforms have greatly expanded our understanding of the mechanism of action of these drugs and allowed further drug development. In keeping with their potent biological activity, meta-analysis suggests that traditional NSAIDs have a valid clinical role as analgesics in cancer pain, as defined by single- and multiple-dose studies. Their efficacy in bone pain however, for which they are frequently prescribed, has not been specifically proven.

The Cox-1 inhibitory activity of NSAIDs is likely to account for several of the adverse effects associated with their use. The identification of a second Cox enzyme (Cox-2), induced under conditions of inflammation, raises the possibility of selective inhibition with minimisation of such side-effects. NSAIDs have been ascribed a dual Cox-1 and Cox-2 inhibitory role, with some such as meloxicam being defined as preferential Cox-2 inhibitors on the basis of *in vitro* and *ex vivo* studies. How well such assays reflect *in vivo* activity is controversial, and has added impetus to the development of the highly specific Cox-2 inhibitors now undergoing phase III clinical trials. However, their clinical efficacy in cancer pain is as yet unproven, and experimental models suggest residual potential for significant GI and renal adverse effects. Further clinical trials are needed to clarify these issues and define the most appropriate roles for 'old' versus 'new' NSAIDs in cancer pain.

References

Bjorkman R (1995). Central antinociceptive effects of non-steroidal anti-inflammatory drugs and paracetamol. *Acta Anaesthesiol Scand* **39**(Suppl.103), 1–44.
Cannon G, Caldwell J & Holt P (1998). MK-0966, a specific Cox-2 inhibitor, has clinical efficacy similar to diclofenac in the treatment of knee and hip osteoarthritis (OA) in a 2-week controlled clinical trial. *Arthritis Rheum* **40**(Suppl.9), S83.

Carlsson K-H, Mangel W & Jurna I (1988). Depression by morphine and the non-opioid analgesic agents, metamizol (dipyrone), lysine acetylsalicylate and paracetamol, of activity in rat thalamus neurones by electrical stimulation of nociceptive afferents. *Pain* **32**, 313–26.

Cashman JN (1996). The mechanism of action of NSAIDs in analgesia. *Drugs* **52**(Suppl.5), 13–23.

Coles LS, Fries JF, Kraines KG & Roth SH (1983). From experiment to experience, side effects of nonsteroidal anti-inflammatory drugs. *Am J Med* **74**, 820–8.

Copeland RA, Williams JN, Giannaras J, Nurnberg S, Covington M, Pinto D, Pick S & Tazaskos JM (1994). Mechanism of selective inhibition of the inducible isoform of prostaglandin G/H synthase. *Proc Natl Acad Sci USA* **91**, 11202–6.

Dequeker J, Hawkey C, Kahan A, Steinbruck K, Alegre C *et al.* on behalf of the SELECT Study Group (1998). Improvement in gastrointestinal tolerability of the selective cyclooxygenase (Cox)-2 inhibitor meloxicam, compared with peroxicam; results of the safety and efficacy large scale evaluation of cox-inhibiting therapies (SELECT) trial in osteoarthritis. *Br J Rheum* **37**, 946–51.

Devoghel J-C (1983). Small intrathecal doses of lysine-acetylsalicylate relieve intractable pain in man. *J Int Med Res* **11**, 90–1.

Douthwaite AH & Lintott SAM (1938). Gastroscopic observation of the effect of aspirin and certain other substances on the stomach. *Lancet* **2**, 1222–5.

Dray A (1995). Inflammatory mediators and pain. *Br J Anaesth* **75**, 125–31.

Dreser H (1899). Pharmacologisches Über Aspirin (acetylsalicyl-saüre). *Pflugers Arch* **76**, 306–18.

Eisenberg E, Berkey CS, Carr DB, Mosteller F & Chalmers TC (1994). Efficacy and safety of nonsteroidal antiinflammatory drugs for cancer pain, a meta-analysis. *J Clin Oncol* **12**, 2756–65.

Ellrich J, Schepelmann K, Pawlak M & Messlinger K (1999). Acetylsalicylic acid inhibits meningeal nociception in rat. *Pain* **81**, 7–14.

Gabriel SE, Jaakkimainen L & Bombardier C (1991). Risk for serious gastrointestinal complications related to use of nonsteroidal anti-inflammatory drugs. A meta-analysis. *Annals Int Med* **115**, 787–96.

Garcia Rodriguez LA & Jick H (1994). Risk of upper gastrointestinal bleeding and perforation associated with individual non-steroidal anti-inflammatory drugs. *Lancet* **343**, 769–72.

Garner A (1992). Adaptation in the pharmaceutical industry, with particular reference to gastrointestinal drugs and diseases. *Scand J Gastroenterol* **27**(Suppl.193), 83–9.

Gretzer B, Knorth H, Chantrain M, Barbera L, Willberger RE, Wittenberg RH & Peskar BM (1998). Effects of diclofenac and L-745,337, a selective cyclooxygenase-2 inhibitor, on prostaglandin E2 formation in tissue from human colonic mucosa and chronic bursitis. *Gastroenterology* **114**, A139.

Harris RC, McKenna JA, Akai Y, Jacobson HR, Dubois RN & Breyer MD (1994). Cyclooxygenase-2 is associated with the macula densa of rat kidney and increases with salt restriction. *J Clin Invest* **94**, 2504–10.

Hawkey C (1999). Cox-2 inhibitors. *Lancet* **353**, 307–14.

Herschman HR (1996). Prostaglandin synthase-2. *Biochim Biophys Acta* **1299**, 125–40.

Herschman HR (1998). Recent progress in the cellular and molecular biology of prostaglandin synthesis. *Trends Cardiovasc Med* **8**, 145–50.

Hosie J, Distel M & Bluhmki E (1998). Meloxicam in osteoarthritis; a six month, double blind comparison with diclofenac sodium. *Br J Rheum* **35**(Suppl.), 39–43.

Hubbard RC, Geiss GS, Woods EM, Yu JS & Zhao W (1998). Efficacy, tolerability and safety of celecoxib, a specific Cox-2 inhibitor, in osteoarthritis. *Rheumatol Eur* **27**(Suppl.1), 118.

Jurna I, Spohrer B & Bock R (1992). Intrathecal injection of acetylsalicyclic acid, salicylic acid and indomethicin depresses C-evoked activity in the rat thalamus and spinal cord. *Pain* **49**, 249–56.

Kawai S, Nishida S, Kato M, Furumaya Y, Okamoto R, Koshino T & Mizushima Y (1998). Comparison of cyclooxygenase-1 and -2 activities of various nonsteroidal anti-inflammatory drugs using human platelets and synovial cells. *European J Pharmacol* **347**, 87–94.

Koch M, Dozi A, Ferrario F & Capurso L (1996). Prevention of nonsteroidal anti-inflammatory drug-induced gastrointestinal mucosal injury; a meta-analysis of randomised controlled clinical trials. *Archives Int Med* **156**, 2321–32.

Langenbach R, Morham SG, Tiano HF, Loftin CD, Ghanaem BI, Chulada PC, Mahler JF, Lee CA, Goulding EH, Kluckman KD, Kim HS & Smithies O (1995). Prostaglandin synthase 1 gene disruption in mice reduces arachidonic acid-induced inflammation and indomethicin-induced gastric ulceration. *Cell* **83**, 483–92.

Langman MJS, Weil J, Wainwright P, Lawsin DH, Rawlins MD, Logan RFA, Murphy M, Vessey MP & Colin-Jones DG (1994). Risks of bleeding peptic ulcer associated with individual non-steroidal anti-inflammatory drugs. *Lancet* **343**, 1075–8.

Lanza FL (1989). A review of gastric ulcer and gastroduodenal injury in normal volunteers receiving aspirin and other nonsteroidal anti-inflammatory drugs. *Scand J Gastroenterol* **24**(Suppl.63), 24–31.

Lanzo CA, Beechem JM, Talley J & Marnett LJ (1998). Investigation of the binding of isoform-selective inhibitors to prostaglandin endoperoxide synthases using fluorescence spectroscopy. *Biochemistry* **37**, 217–26.

Loll PJ, Picot D & Garavito RM (1995). The structural basis of aspirin activity inferred from the crystal structure of inactivated prostaglandin H_2 synthase. *Nature Struct Biol* **2**, 637–42.

Luong C, Miller A, Barnett J, Chow J, Ramasha C & Browner MF (1996). The structure of human cyclooxygenase-2; conservation and flexibility of the NSAID binding site. *Nat Struct Biol* **3**, 927–33.

McCormack K (1994). Non-steroidal anti-inflammatory drugs and spinal nociceptive processing. *Pain* **59**, 9–43.

MacDonald TM, Morant SV & Robinson GC (1997). Association of upper gastrointestinal toxicity of non-steroidal anti-inflammatory drugs with continued exposure. *BMJ* **315**, 1333–7.

McGoldrick MD & Bailie GR (1997). Nonnarcotic analgesics, prevalence and estimated economic impact of toxicities. *Ann Pharmacother* **31**, 245–8.

Mamberg AB & Yaksh TL (1992). Hyperalgesia mediated by spinal glutamate or substance P receptor blocked by spinal cyclooxygenase inhibition. *Science* **257**, 1276–9.

Mancini JA, Riendeau D, Falgueyret JP, Vickers PJ & O'Neill GP (1995). Arginine 120 of prostaglandin G/H synthase-1 is required for the inhibition by nonsteroidal anti-inflammatory drugs containing a carboxylic acid moiety. *J Biol Chem* **270**, 29372–7.

Mariolo N, Ehrlich K, Schuligoi R, Respondek M & Peskar BM (1998). Cyclooxygenase-2 derived prostaglandins contribute to mucosal resistence to ischaemia/reperfusion injury in the rat stomach. *Gastroenterology* **114**, A215.

Møller Hansen J, Hallas J, Lauritsen JM & Dytzer P (1996). Non-steroidal anti-inflammatory drugs and ulcer complications; a risk factor analysis for clinical decision making. *Scand J Gastroenterol* **31**, 126–30.

Moreham SG, Langenbach R, Loftin CD, Tiano HF, Vouloumanos N, Jeanette JC, Mahler JF, Kluckman KD, Ledford A, Lee CA & Smithies O (1995). Prostaglandin synthase 2 gene disruption causes severe renal pathology in the mouse. *Cell* **83**, 473–82.

Murray MD, Brater DC, Tierney WM, Hui SL & McDonald CJ (1990). Ibuprofen-associated renal impairment in a large general internal medicine practice. *Am J Med Sci* **299**, 222–9.

Noble S & Balfour JA (1996). Meloxicam. *Drugs* **51**, 424–32.

Palmer BF (1995). Renal complications associated with the use of nonsteroidal anti-inflammatory agents. *J Invest Med* **43**, 516–33.

Picot D, Loll PJ & Garavito RM (1994). The x-ray crystal structure of the membrane protein prostaglandin H2 synthase-1. *Nature* **367**, 243–9.

Reuter BK, Asfaha S, Buret A, Sharkey KA & Wallace JL (1996). Exacerbation of inflammation-associated colonic injury in rat through inhibition of cyclooxygenase-2. *J Clin Invest* **98**, 2076–85.

Rostom A, Welch V, Wells G, Tugwell P, Dubæ C, Lanas A & McGowan J (1999). Prostaglandin analogues, H2 receptor antagonists and proton pump inhibitors for the prevention of chronic NSAID induced upper gastrointestinal toxicity in adults: protocol. *Cochrane Library* Issue 2, Update Software, Oxford.

Service RF (1996). Closing in on a stomach sparing aspirin. *Science* **273**, 1660.

Stoll BA (1973). Indomethicin in breast cancer. *Lancet* **ii**, 384.

Takahasi S, Shigeta J, Kobayasi N & Okabe S (1998). Localization of cyclooxygenase-2 and regulation of its expression in gastric ulcer in rats. *Gastroenterology* **114**, A303.

Vane JR (1971). Inhibition of prostaglandin synthesis as a mechanism of action for aspirin-like drugs. *Nature New Biol* **231**, 232–5.

Vane JR (1994). Towards a better aspirin. *Nature* **367**, 215–16.

Wallace JL (1997). Non-steroidal anti-inflammatory drugs and gastroenteropathy, the second hundred years. *Gastroenterology* **112**, 1000–16.

Wallace JR, Bak A, McKnight W, Asfaha S, Sharkey KA & McNaughton WK (1998). Cyclooxygenase 1 contributes to inflammatory responses in rats and mice; implications for gastrointestinal toxicity. *Gastroenterology* **115**, 101–9.

World Health Organization (1986). *Cancer pain relief.* WHO, Geneva, Switzerland.

Xie W, Chipman JG, Robertson DL, Erikson RL & Simmons DL (1991). Expression of a mitogen-responsive gene encoding prostaglandin synthase is regulated by mRNA splicing. *Proc Natl Acad Sci USA* **88**, 2692–6.

Chapter 8

Central issues in the management of temporal variation in cancer pain

IAC Douglas, L Wilson and RF Lennard

Introduction

The concept of cancer pain being constant and unrelenting has served patients well. It is one of the concepts on which 'around the clock' (ATC) dose scheduling is based, which in turn is one the central themes of many of the cancer pain management guidelines. Researchers who have assessed the effectiveness of the World Health Organization (WHO) guidelines have concluded that compliance with them leads to acceptable pain control in between 70 and 90 per cent of patients (Ventafridda *et al.* 1987). This means that somewhere between 10 and 30 per cent of patients do not achieve good control of their pain using the opioid ladder combined with adjuvant non-steroidal anti-inflammatory drugs (NSAIDs), as appropriate.

Anecdotally, clinicians recognise that one factor that may predict failure to achieve good analgesic control is temporal variation in the severity of a patient's pain. Bruera *et al.* (1995) and Mercadante *et al.* (1992) have shown that the presence of 'incident pain' predicts a poor response to analgesics. Banning *et al.* (1991) highlighted the difficulty in providing pain relief to those patients who had pain on motion related to bone metastases. This realisation has meant that temporal variation in cancer pain has attracted significant interest in recent years.

In this chapter, we will describe some of the research on the prevalence of these pains that vary in intensity, and the trends in their management. First, however, we need to introduce the terminology used in the field.

Terminology

The terminology used to describe temporal variation in cancer pain has been evolving over the last ten years and remains confusing (McQuay & Jadad 1994; Portenoy 1997; Patt & Ellison 1998). The following terms have been used.

- *Breakthrough pain* – to many clinicians 'breakthrough' implies that the patient is already on a regular ATC analgesic regimen and that the basal pain is already controlled by that regimen. Portenoy & Hagen's (1990) initial research definition was 'a transitory exacerbation of pain that occurs on a background of otherwise stable pain in a patient receiving chronic opioid therapy'. Portenoy (1997) later enlarged the definition to include patients not on analgesics ('transitory increases in pain that occur in patients with chronic baseline pain'). More recently, he has specified that such increases are directly related to the background pain (Portenoy *et al.* 1999a). Other researchers and clinicians have used 'breakthrough pain' as an umbrella term under which other terms are placed. 'Breakthrough pain' is a useful text phrase with which to search databases for papers on pain that varies with time.

- *Incident pain* – the most commonly held understanding of this term in the UK is 'episodes of pain related to movement'. McQuay & Jadad (1994), in their review of incident pain, define it as 'pain that comes on when the patient is not resting'. However, they go on to suggest that the simplest possible definition would include all episodic increases in pain intensity with or without a triggering process. This definition would include breakthrough pains as described above and, for instance, intermittent neuropathic pains with no stimulus. In contrast, Portenoy suggests that incident pain may be considered to be a subtype of breakthrough pain.

- *End-of-dose pain* – this describes pain that occurs only near to the time when the next dose of analgesia is due. The implication is that the level of analgesia has fallen to a subtherapeutic level before the next ATC dose is due.

- *Episodic pain* – this term has been used by several authors either interchangeably with breakthrough pain (Hanks *et al.* 1998) or as a broad term under which breakthrough pain, incident pain and end-of-dose pain exist (Coluzzi 1998).

- *Recurrent acute pain* – Portenoy distinguishes recurrent acute pain from breakthrough pain in that recurrent acute pain does *not* occur against a background of similar pain (Portenoy *et al.* 1999a).

We have elected to use 'episodic pain' as an umbrella term in this chapter. We define the phenomenon as any discrete and recurring episodes of pain that are time-limited and can occur with or without a similar baseline steady pain at the same location. The term used in this context includes 'breakthrough pain', 'incident pain', 'end-of-dose pain' and 'recurrent acute pain'.

Prevalence

The prevalence of episodic pains has been studied in a variety of cancer patient populations who have either been referred to specialist palliative care or pain services or been admitted to cancer treatment centres. As yet there have been no studies in the general cancer patient population. The main studies are listed in Box 8.1, with some description of the different patient groups and types of episodic pain measured.

It is not possible to compare these studies directly because the researchers have classified the temporal variations in pain in different ways. However, it is clear that episodic pains are common in patients referred to specialist palliative care and pain services, and in these selected populations, may be commoner than the steady continuous pains traditionally associated with cancer.

Aetiology, pathophysiology and characteristics

In the studies described above the authors have used a variety of assessment schedules, the most common being that created by Portenoy & Hagen (1990). Most have asked patients to recall episodes of pain in the previous 24 hours and to rate their frequency, duration and intensity of exacerbation and sometimes their impact on function. These studies have also variously described the aetiology and pathophysiology of the episodes of pain they have recorded.

Aetiology

Some authors have categorised their episodic pains into the four categories of cancer pain described by Twycross (1982), i.e. pain caused by direct cancer involvement, pain caused by cancer treatment, pain associated with cancer-related debility and pain unrelated to the patient's cancer or its treatment.

Portenoy & Hagen (1990) found that 82 per cent of their 'breakthrough pains' were directly caused by or associated with the cancer, 14 per cent were related to treatment and 4 per cent were unrelated to the cancer or its treatment. Similarly, Banning et al. (1991), in their population with a large proportion of incident pains, found 61 per cent of all pains recorded were directly caused by the cancer, 6 per cent were related to treatment, 25 per cent were associated with cancer debility and 8 per cent were unrelated to the cancer or to treatment. These figures approximate to Grond's findings concerning the aetiology of *all* cancer pains (Grond et al. 1996). From this limited evidence it seems likely that episodic pains have similar aetiologies to all pains in cancer patients.

Pathophysiology

Most of the studies have classified the episodic pains that they have recorded under the broad headings of somatic pain, visceral pain, neuropathic pain and mixed pain. The ranges of proportions of each type of pain found are: somatic (33–46 per cent); visceral (20–30 per cent); neuropathic (10–27 per cent); and mixed (16–20 per cent) (Portenoy & Hagen 1990; Zech et al. 1995; Zeppetella et al. personal communication). The prevalence of these pathophysiological types is again similar to that described by Grond et al. (1996) for all pain syndromes in cancer patients.

Box 8.1

- Portenoy & Hagen (1990) assessed 90 inpatients referred to their pain service over a three-month period. Sixty-three of the patients met their requirements of stable opioid dosage for the previous 48 hours and baseline pain of moderate or less intensity. In this selected group, 63 per cent described one or more episodes in the previous 24 hours of severe or excruciating pain (breakthrough pain). Twenty-eight per cent had more than one distinct type of breakthrough pain.

- Portenoy et al. (1999a) recently repeated this initial study in an inpatient population of cancer patients within an oncology treatment centre and found 51 per cent had experienced breakthrough pain in the previous 24 hours.

- Banning et al. (1991) analysed pain in 200 consecutive cancer referrals to a pain clinic. The median survival of the group was ten weeks. Although not focusing specifically on episodic pain, their results show that 86 per cent of the patients had pain on motion. Those with bone pain on movement formed a particularly difficult group to treat.

- Zech et al. (1995) studied 613 cancer patients referred to their pain clinic. They defined breakthrough pain as any pain that is 'characterised by transience and intensity over baseline'. Using this definition, 40 per cent had breakthrough pain.

- Fine & Busch (1998) studied 22 terminally ill patients with pain at home. Eighty-six per cent had breakthrough pain using Portenoy's definition.

- Grond et al. (1996) assessed 2,266 new referrals with cancer pain to their pain service and classified their pain using the IASP classification of chronic pain (International Association for the Study of Pain 1986). Axis III of the classification divides the temporal characteristic of any pain into nine categories. They found 23 per cent of the main pain syndromes were classified as 'recurring regularly or irregularly', 'paroxysmal' or 'sustained with paroxysms'. A further 36 per cent were classified as 'continuous, fluctuating'.

- Zeppetella, O'Doherty & Collins (personal communication) prospectively surveyed pain patterns in 414 consecutive hospice admissions using a schedule adapted from Portenoy & Hagen (1990). Of those with pain, 89 per cent described one or more breakthrough pains.

- Swanwick, Haworth & Lennard (personal communication) studied 132 hospice admissions who had experienced 228 separate pains in the previous 24 hours. Only 7 per cent of these were steady continuous pains. The remaining 93 per cent varied with time, 36 per cent having a background element (corresponding approximately to Portenoy's 'breakthrough pains') and 57 per cent occurring in the absence of any background pain (recurrent, acute pains).

Temporal characteristics

There are several different temporal characteristics of episodic pains which have been described. First, there is the time from the onset of the pain to its peak intensity, second, the duration of the episode and lastly the frequency with which the episodes of pain occur. These characteristics have been recorded by Zech *et al.* (1995), Portenoy & Hagen (1990), Zeppetella *et al.* (personal communication) and Swanwick *et al.* (personal communication). Typically, they find the time period of onset to peak intensity to be less than three minutes in about half of their patients (range 43–55 per cent). The mean and median durations of the episodes of episodic pain are about 30 minutes. The range of mean and median frequencies of episodes was 7–10 and 2–4 per day respectively.

Intensity and impact

These are not trivial pains. All of Portenoy & Hagen's were, by definition, severe to excruciating. In a recent paper, Portenoy *et al.* (1999a) have shown that the presence of breakthrough pain independently contributes to a patient's impaired functioning and psychological distress. Zech *et al.* (1995) found a mean pain score of 4.9/10 for their episodic pains. Fine & Busch (1998) found a mean score of 7/10 for the episodic pains of their patients at home. Zeppetella *et al.* (personal communication) found 38 per cent of the episodic pains in hospice admissions were severe to excruciating. Swanwick *et al.* (personal communication), also in hospice admissions, found a median pain score of 8/10 for episodes of pain on top of background pain and 6/10 for episodes of pain with no background. Of these pains, 36 per cent were completely incapacitating when they occurred. Coyle *et al.* (1990) describe a 'difficult' group of cancer pain patients during their last four weeks of life. They found that 39 per cent of patients with average pain varying between mild and moderate described incident pain (definition used – 'pain following a voluntary act, usually movement') as a major limiting factor to activity. Of those patients with moderate-to-severe average pain, 94 per cent described incident pain as a major limitation to activity.

Precipitants

Portenoy & Hagen (1990) found that 55 per cent of their patients' breakthrough pains had precipitants, of which 78 per cent were volitional. Grond *et al.* (1996) assessed a subgroup of their patients and found that 69 per cent had precipitants for their pain. For 38 per cent, the precipitant was movement or walking. Fine & Busch (1998) found about half of their patients' breakthrough pains had definite precipitants.

Relationship of breakthrough pain to background pain

A judgement can be made clinically as to whether the episode of pain is an exacerbation of the continuous pain or whether it is qualitatively different. The latter implies that the episodic pain may have a different pathophysiology from that of the background pain. Authors have come to different conclusions. Portenoy & Hagen (1990) found that 96 per cent of 'breakthrough' pains were in the same location as baseline pains and were recognised as being directly related to the background pain. McQuay & Jadad (1994) suggest that 'incident' pain may be qualitatively different from pain at rest, often being neuropathic in nature.

Acute, recurring pains may truly have no background component, or the background pain may have been masked by regular analgesia, leaving only the exacerbations evident. It is not clear, therefore, from the research studies so far, that acute, recurring pains form a different group from pains with exacerbations on a background of continuous pain.

Summary

Episodic pains do not form a homogenous group, but overall they have a considerable impact on those who experience them. Pain on movement forms the largest definable subgroup. Clinical experience would suggest that bone pain on weight bearing or movement forms a majority of pain in this subgroup, but this has not been demonstrated in research to date.

Management

When McQuay & Jadad (1994) undertook their review of incident pain, they could not find any reports of randomised controlled trials of 'incident' pain management in cancer patients despite using a sophisticated search strategy. There now exists some research into the management of 'breakthrough' pain, which we review below. In the literature, three main strategies have been suggested once disease-altering treatment has been exhausted (McQuay & Jadad 1994; Portenoy 1997; Patt & Ellison 1998). These are reviewed below.

To address the pathophysiological cause

There are well-recognised clinical syndromes that lead to episodic pain in cancer patients. Many of these pains are traditionally thought to be less responsive to opioid analgesia than continuous cancer pain. Their responsiveness to either ATC opioids or rescue doses of opioids should be assessed but their pathophysiological mechanism can also be directly targeted. Table 8.1 lists these syndromes together with treatment strategies that are commonly tried. There are very few clinical trials to support these approaches but many are now widely accepted as current best practice and are recommended in standard palliative medicine textbooks (e.g. Doyle et al. 1998; Twycross 1994, 1997).

To optimise the response to opioids

The rationale of this approach is the assumption that most episodic pains are an exacerbation of continuous cancer pain. If the continuous cancer pain is opioid-

Table 8.1 Accepted management strategies for common episodic pains in cancer patients

Pain	Management strategy
Neuropathic pain	Tricyclic antidepressants, anticonvulsants, Class 1 antiarrhythmics, steroids
Abdominal colic	Anticholinergic drugs (e.g. amitriptyline, buscopan, cyclizine), mebeverine, octreotide
Bladder spasm	Anticholinergic drugs (e.g. amitriptyline, oxybutinin, flavoxate), NSAIDs
Tenesmoid pain	Nifedipine, sympathetic nerve block, local or systemic steroids or treat as neuropathic pain as above
Pleuritic pain	NSAIDs, steroids, local anaesthetic (intrapleural infusions, paravertebral block, intercostal nerve block)
Oesophageal spasm	Nifedipine, antifungals (if candidiasis suspected)
Skeletal muscle spasm	Baclofen, dantrolene, benzodiazepines
Bone pain on movement	Radiotherapy, NSAIDs, steroids, bisphosphonates, surgical fixation, immobilisation
Pain assoc. with procedures	Nitrous oxide, ketamine, benzodiazepine sedation (special consideration should be given to the use of short acting opioids)

responsive, the problem then becomes how to achieve adequate plasma levels of opioid to control the exacerbation without suffering unnecessary adverse effects when the pain level is less.

As discussed previously, the onset of episodic pains is often abrupt and their duration short. Clearly, what is required in the above situation are opioids with rapid onset and short duration of action and an appropriate delivery system to allow them to be used in clinical practice. Current guidelines suggest that patients should be instructed to take a fixed dose of an immediate-release preparation of oral opioid usually after the onset of an episode of pain. This extra dose is referred to as 'rescue analgesia' or sometimes 'breakthrough analgesia'.

In contrast to the abruptness of onset of most episodic pains, the onset of analgesia for most of the orally administered opioids is greater than 30 minutes. This time required to achieve analgesia is consistent with pharmacokinetic studies which show the plasma T(max) of orally administered morphine and oxycodone are both about 45 minutes (Osbourne *et al.* 1990; Poyhia *et al.* 1992). Again, in contrast to the short duration of most episodic pains, the duration of action of most orally administered opioids is three or more hours; this may result in unwanted sedation once the episode of pain has resolved.

Possible future developments

Recently, therefore, clinicians have looked at opioids which are rapidly absorbed by mouth and have a short duration of action. Oral transmucosal fentanyl citrate (OTFC) fits this description. Pharmacokinetic studies have shown that the T(max) for OTFC is 22 minutes (Streisand *et al.*1991). Time to the onset of analgesic action in one study was in the region of ten minutes (Fine *et al.* 1991); in another, two-thirds of pain relief was achieved within 15 minutes (Christie *et al.* 1998; Simmonds 1997). There is now a significant body of published research related to the use of OTFC in the management of episodic cancer pain (Cleary 1997; Coluzzi 1997; Lyss 1997; Portenoy *et al.* 1999b). Unwanted opioid effects were recorded as mild and predictable in nature in all the studies. A preparation of OTFC has now been given Food and Drug Administration (FDA) approval for breakthrough pain in cancer patients receiving strong opioids.

Fentanyl has also been used intranasally (Striebel *et al.* 1993). The majority of experience in its use has been in the post-operative setting (Striebel *et al.* 1996) but there are case reports of intranasal fentanyl use in patients with pain related to metastatic cancer (O'Neil *et al.* 1997). Zeppetella (personal communication) has performed an open study of the use of intranasal fentanyl in the management of breakthrough pain in cancer. The results from this study are encouraging but need to be confirmed in randomised trials. An intranasal delivery device for fentanyl and pethidine has been developed and licensed in Australia (Go Medical, Australia).

The use of a rescue dose of oral analgesia as described above is, in effect, oral patient-controlled analgesia (PCA). Patients are given control over their own analgesia in order to shorten the time between their experiencing pain and receiving adequate analgesia. In other areas of clinical practice the onset of analgesia is further shortened by delivering opioids intravenously. There is significant evidence from these areas of practice that intravenous PCA is effective, safe and preferred by patients. There have, however, been no large studies of its use for patients with chronic cancer pain. The physical inconvenience of the equipment required is significant and, until recently, the cost of the devices has been prohibitive. There are now cheaper disposable devices available but it seems unlikely that intravenous PCA will enter routine practice in the care of patients with chronic cancer pain, despite the pharmacokinetic advantages of this route for the treatment of episodic pain.

There is evidence in children that onset of analgesic action following subcutaneous injection is comparable to intravenous injection for lipophylic drugs (Doyle *et al.* 1994). Since the subcutaneous route is more easily maintained in a domiciliary setting, subcutaneous PCA could be considered if a parenteral route for PCA is needed.

Other quick-onset and short-acting opioids exist but have not routinely been used to manage cancer pain. In the context of episodic pain, remifentanil is potentially of interest. It differs from other opioids in that it is metabolised by tissue and plasma esterases and therefore has an extremely short duration of action. The potential therefore exists to match the duration of analgesia almost exactly to the duration of the episode of pain. As yet, experience with this drug has been only in the anaesthetic setting.

Finally, the alternative to using short-acting opioids is actively to manage the unwanted effects that occur when the ATC opioid dose is increased. Bruera *et al.* (1992) attempted to do this by using methylphenidate in a group of patients with incident cancer pain. They achieved a significant reduction in mean pain and sedation scores following the addition of methylphenidate 25 mg daily in a divided dose. They were able to increase the mean equivalent daily dose of morphine twofold but do not comment whether the incident component of the patients' pain was improved.

To use a multimodal approach

This approach is modelled on the current approach to the management of post-operative pain (McQuay & Jadad, 1994). In the post-operative setting a significant proportion of the pain experienced is episodic in nature. Episodes of pain are commonly related to movement, coughing and deep breathing. Pain during these activities is now routinely used as outcome measures in post-operative pain control studies. There is general agreement that the use of a multimodal analgesic approach improves post-operative pain control (Agency for Health Care Policy and Research 1992; Kehlet & Dahl 1993; Hopf & Weitz 1994). The term 'multimodal' implies the use of several analgesic drugs delivered by a number of different routes. A patient may, for instance, receive pre-emptive treatment with steroids and opioids pre-operatively, peri-operative spinal analgesia using opioids and local anaesthetics, and postoperative spinal infusion as well as intravenous PCA. Several authors have concluded that the use of the epidural route is the one independent factor that influences the control of postoperative movement related pain (Kehlet & Dahl 1993; Lynch *et al.* 1997).

Whether this experience is transferable to the setting of episodic cancer pain is unknown. Some evidence comes from two retrospective studies on the use of long-term intrathecal analgesia in patients with inadequately controlled cancer pain (Sjoberg *et al.* 1991; van Dongen *et al.* 1993). These two papers report good or better pain control in 96 and 86 per cent of patients, respectively. It is reasonable to assume from the studies discussed previously (Banning *et al.* 1991; Mercadante *et al.* 1992; Bruera *et al.* 1995) that a significant number of these patients had episodic pain. Further studies are needed to compare this approach to routine practice and to focus on the episodic component of this group of patients' pain.

Measurement in research

There now exists good evidence from studies in various cancer patient populations that episodic pain is common and clinically important. Its management would merit further research. First, however, we need practical, valid, reliable and sensitive pain assessment tools that can assess the impact of treatment strategies on episodic pain as a separate entity from background pain. Pain intensity and pain affect (the perceived unpleasantness of the pain) have been shown to respond differentially to interventions in movement-related pain as well as continuous pain (Smith *et al.* 1998). Outcome measures should therefore include pain affect and patient preference as well as pain intensity and pain relief. Change in the impact of episodic pain on patients' lives should also be assessed. Portenoy *et al.* (1999a) included many of these measures in their recent prevalence study, but this approach has not yet been applied to intervention studies.

There are other areas of clinical practice where episodic pain is common and where pain assessment tools have been developed. For instance, it is now standard in post-operative pain studies to assess pain intensity during specific activities such as deep breathing, coughing or moving from lying to sitting. Similarly, researchers into pain associated with osteoarthritis have developed a tool which evaluates episodic pain related to activities of daily living (Rejeski *et al.* 1995). Known as the 'knee pain scale', it measures both the frequency and intensity of pain experienced during walking and transferring. It appears to be a good model against which to create similar scales for specific subgroups of cancer patients with episodic pain provoked by activity.

Much of pain research has relied on remembered pain intensity and relief scores. We do not know whether this approach is valid for episodes of pain in the clinical setting (Erskine *et al.* 1990). Many factors, including current pain intensity, current mood and beliefs about pain aetiology, influence remembered pain scores (Smith *et al.* 1998). Dependence on remembered scores can be avoided by undertaking numerous contemporaneous scores. Portenoy *et al.* (1999b) took this approach in their study of the use of OTFC for breakthrough pain. Their patients made multiple recordings of pain intensity and relief during episodes of breakthrough pain. Electronic data loggers are now available and may make this approach more practical.

Future research

The prevalence studies of episodic pain have demonstrated the unexpectedly common problem of pains for which the usual regular doses of long acting opioids are not appropriate. These pains merit some further analysis and classification; their discovery should stimulate research into their management.

Potential areas of research might include the following:

- a comparison of increasing the dose of ATC opioid analgesia with the optimal use of short-acting opioid rescue analgesia;
- further investigation of the targeted use of short-acting opioids linked with PCA systems;
- the management of opioid-related side-effects to allow opioid dose escalation;
- defining the role of radiotherapy, NSAIDs, bisphosphonates and internal fixation in the management of episodic bone pain on movement and weight bearing;
- the role of spinal analgesia in the management of episodic pain;
- assessment of the benefit of tricyclic antidepressants and old and new anticonvulsants in the management of neuropathic pain.

Conclusion

Prevalence studies of episodic pain in specialist pain and palliative care centres have revealed an unexpectedly large number of cancer patients with pain that varies significantly with time. These pains do not all respond to regular opioid analgesia and adjuvant drugs titrated according to WHO guidelines.

This finding has stimulated research into the use of short-acting opioids, such as oral transmucosal fentanyl citrate, for the treatment of 'breakthrough pain', and results of their effectiveness seem promising. However, episodic pains do not form a homogenous group and it would be helpful to further define subgroups with similar aetiologies in order to focus on management based on the pathophysiological basis of the pain. The presence of episodic pain is often one feature of complex cancer pain syndromes and a multimodal approach to pain control may be necessary to obtain good pain relief. All research in this area would be made easier by agreement on reliable measurement tools and consistent terminology.

The work so far in this field challenges us to think differently about our treatment of a significant proportion of cancer pains. Large numbers of cancer patients will benefit if we can improve our management of those pains that vary with time.

Acknowledgements

The authors are members of the Yorkshire Palliative Medicine Training Rotation Research Group. Many of the papers cited in this chapter were found by other members' painstaking searches. We are grateful to them for these and for their comments on early drafts of this chapter.

Marie Curie have generously funded Rosemary Lennard to facilitate and supervise this research group – without their help the group would not have progressed to the point of writing such a chapter.

Janssen-Cilag's contribution to the running expenses of the group has funded the literature search and acquisition of the references.

References

Agency for Health Care Policy and Research (1992). Acute pain management: operative or medical procedures and trauma, Part 2. AHCPR [Review] [279 refs]. *Clinical Pharmacy* **11**, 391–414.

Banning A, Sjogren P & Henriksen H (1991). Pain causes in 200 patients referred to a multidisciplinary cancer pain clinic. *Pain* **45**, 45–8.

Bruera E, Fainsinger R., MacEachern T & Hanson J (1992). The use of methylphenidate in patients with incident cancer pain receiving regular opiates. A preliminary report. *Pain* **50**, 75–7.

Bruera E, Schoeller T, Wenk R, MacEachern T, Marcelino, Hanson J & Suarez-Almazor M (1995). A prospective multicenter assessment of the Edmonton staging system for cancer pain. *Journal of Pain & Symptom Management* **10**, 348–55.

Christie JM, Simmonds M, Patt R, Coluzzi P, Busch MA, Nordbrock E & Portenoy RK (1998). Dose-titration, multicenter study of oral transmucosal fentanyl citrate for the treatment of breakthrough pain in cancer patients using transdermal fentanyl for persistent pain. *J Clin Oncol* **16**, 3238–45.

Cleary JF (1997). Double blind randomised study of the treatment of breakthrough pain in cancer patients: oral transmucosal fentanyl citrate versus placebo. *Proceedings of ASCO* **16**, 52a (Abstract).

Coluzzi P (1997). A titration study of oral transmucosal fentanyl citratefor breakthrough pain in cancer patients. *Proceedings of ASCO* **16**, 41a (Abstract).

Coluzzi PH (1998). Cancer pain management: newer perspectives on opioids and episodic pain [Review] [20 refs]. *American Journal of Hospice & Palliative Care* **15**, 13–22.

Coyle N, Adelhardt J, Foley KM & Portenoy RK (1990). Character of terminal illness in the advanced cancer patient: Pain and other symptoms during the last four weeks of life. *Journal of Pain & Symptom Management* **5**, 83–93.

Doyle D, Hanks GWC & MacDonald N (eds) (1998). *Oxford textbook of palliative medicine* 2nd edn. Oxford University Press, New York.

Doyle E, Norton NS & McNicol LR (1994). Comparison of patient-controlled analgesia in children by i.v. and s.c. routes of administration. *British Journal of Anaesthesia* **72**, 533–6.

Erskine A, Morley S & Pearce S (1990). Memory for pain: a review [Review] [35 refs]. *Pain* **41**, 255–65.

Fine PG & Busch MA (1998). Characterization of breakthrough pain by hospice patients and their caregivers. *Journal of Pain & Symptom Management* **16**, 179–83.

Fine PG, Marcus M, De Boer AJ & Van der Oord B (1991). An open label study of oral transmucosal fentanyl citrate (OTFC) for the treatment of breakthrough cancer pain. *Pain* **45**, 149–53.

Grond S, Zech D, Diefenbach C, Radbruch L & Lehmann KA (1996). Assessment of cancer pain: a prospective evaluation in 2266 cancer patients referred to a pain service. *Pain* **64**, 107–14.

Hanks G, Portenoy RK, MacDonald N & Forbes K (1998). Difficult pain problems. In *Oxford Textbook of Palliative Medicine* (ed. D Doyle, G Hanks & N MacDonald), pp. 454–77. Oxford University Press, New York

Hopf HW & Weitz S (1994). Postoperative pain management [Review] [74 refs]. *Archives of Surgery* **129**, 128–32.

IASP (1986). Classification of chronic pain. *Pain* (Suppl.3), 1–226.

Kehlet H & Dahl JB (1993). The value of 'multimodal' or 'balanced analgesia' in postoperative pain treatment [Review] [92 refs]. *Anesthesia & Analgesia* **77**, 1048–56.

Lynch EP, Lazor MA, Gellis JE, Orav J, Goldman L & Marcantonio ER (1997). Patient experience of pain after elective noncardiac surgery. *Anesthesia & Analgesia* **85**, 117–23.

Lyss A (1997). Long-term use of oral transmucosal fentanyl citrate for breakthrough pain in cancer patients. *Proceedings of ASCO* **16**, 41a (Abstract).

McQuay HJ & Jadad AR (1994). Incident pain. *Cancer Surveys* **21**, 17–24.

Mercadante S, Maddaloni S, Roccella S & Salvaggio L (1992). Predictive factors in advanced cancer pain treated only by analgesics. *Pain* **50**, 151–5.

O'Neil G, Paech M & Wood F (1997). Preliminary clinical use of a patient-controlled intranasal analgesia (PCINA) device. *Anaesthesia & Intensive Care* **25**, 408–12.

Osbourne R, Joel S & Trew D (1990). Morphine and metabolite behaviour after different routes of morphine administration: demonstration of the importance of the active metabolite morphine-6-glucuronide. *Clinical Pharmacology and therapeutics* **47**, 12–19.

Patt RB & Ellison NM (1998). Breakthrough pain in cancer patients: characteristics, prevalence, and treatment [Review] [68 refs]. *Oncology* **12**, 1035–46.

Portenoy RK (1997). Treatment of temporal variations in chronic cancer pain [Review] [16 refs]. *Seminars in Oncology* **24**, S16–12.

Portenoy RK & Hagen NA (1990). Breakthrough pain: definition, prevalence and characteristics [see comments]. *Pain* **41**, 273–81.

Portenoy RK, Payne D & Jacobsen P (1999a). Breakthrough pain: characteristics and impact in patients with cancer pain. *Pain* **81**, 129–34.

Portenoy RK, Payne R, Coluzzi P, Raschko JW, Lyss A, Busch MA, Frigerio V, Ingham J, Loseth DB, Nordbrock E & Rhiner M (1999b). Oral transmucosal fentanyl citrate (OTFC) for the treatment of breakthrough pain in cancer patients: a controlled dose titration study [In Process Citation]. *Pain* **79**, 303–12.

Poyhia R, Seppala T & Olkkola T (1992). The pharmacokinetics and metabolism of oxycodone after intramuscular and oral administration to healthy subjects. *British journal of Clinical Pharmacology* **33**, 617–21.

Rejeski WJ, Ettinger WHJ, Shumaker S, Heuser M D, James P, Monu J & Burns R (1995). The evaluation of pain in patients with knee osteoarthritis: the knee pain scale. *Journal of Rheumatology* **22**, 1124–9.

Simmonds M (1997). Oral transmucosal fentanyl citrate produces pain relief faster than medication typically used for breakthrough pain in cancer patients. *Proceedings of ASCO* **16**, 52a (Abstract).

Sjoberg M, Appelgren L, Einarsson S, Hultman E, Linder L E, Nitescu P & Curelaru I (1991). Long-term intrathecal morphine and bupivacaine in 'refractory' cancer pain. I. Results from the first series of 52 patients. *Acta Anaesthesiologica Scandinavica* **35**, 30–43.

Smith WB, Gracely RH & Safer MA (1998). The meaning of pain: cancer patients' rating and recall of pain intensity and affect. *Pain* **78**, 123–29.

Streisand J B, Varvel JR, Stanski DR, Le Maire L, Ashburn MA, Hague BI, Tarver SD & Stanley TH (1991). Absorption and bioavailability of oral transmucosal fentanyl citrate. *Anesthesiology* **75**, 223–9.

Striebel HW, Olmann T, Spies C & Brummer G (1996). Patient-controlled intranasal analgesia (PCINA) for the management of postoperative pain: a pilot study. *Journal of Clinical Anesthesia* **8**, 4–8.

Striebel HW, Pommerening J & Rieger A (1993). Intranasal fentanyl titration for postoperative pain management in an unselected population. *Anaesthesia* **48**, 753–7.

Twycross R (1982). Pain in far advanced cancer. *Pain* **14**, 303–10.

Twycross R (1994). *Pain relief in advanced cancer* 1st edn. Churchill Livingstone, Edinburgh.

Twycross R (1997). *Symptom management in advanced cancer* 2nd edn. Radcliffe Medical Press, Oxford.

Van Dongen DR, Crul BJ & De Bock BM (1993). Long-term intrathecal infusion of morphine and morphine/bupivacaine mixtures in the treatment of cancer pain: a retrospective analysis of 51 cases. *Pain* **55**, 119–23.

Ventafridda V, Tamburini M, Caraceni A., De Conno F & Naldi F (1987). A validation study of the WHO method for cancer pain relief. *Cancer* **59**, 850–6.

Zech D, Petzke F, Radbruch L & Grond S (1995). Breakthrough pain in cancer patients with chronic pain: Prevalence and characteristics. *British Journal of Anaesthesia* **74** (Abstract).

Chapter 9

The evidence base for surgical intervention in the management of cancer pain

P Declan Carey, Graeme Bailie and Bernadette A Corcoran

Introduction

One of the primary objectives of the modern cancer surgeon is the curative excision of a primary tumour. With advancement in technologies allowing a more accurate assessment of stage of disease, at the outset of treatment, cancer surgeons are now as likely to discuss palliative forms of treatment. This of course means that in operative terms many surgeons now are aware of the need to attempt palliation of symptoms which herald, in particular, the chronic cancer pain syndromes. This may involve, for instance, the use of nerve-sparing techniques. Much can be done by the surgeon in this palliative approach, where older and more invasive surgical techniques such as the neuroablative ones are increasingly being replaced by minimally invasive loco-regional procedures.

   The main area in cancer pain which involves the surgeon is the management of pain associated with bone metastases and pathological fracture. Apart from this area, little evidence in terms of trial data exists to support the use of radical surgical techniques, in particular the older more aggressive neuroablative procedures, in the control of intractable cancer pain. Thus for much of the evidence relating to surgical involvement in cancer pain management we rely on best-practice guidelines.

   The areas in which the surgeon's role is extensive include management of the pain associated with the cancer in its pre-diagnostic or pre-treatment phases. Solid cancers of tubular organs (urothelial, gastrointestinal) can cause obstruction and thus pain. By and large, the organ-specific surgeon will, by resecting the cancer or organ, relieve this pain. As we progress through the diagnosis-to-treatment cycle, there are many situations where initial treatment and diagnostic techniques will cause pain. These pains must be alleviated. Obviously, the pain induced by any surgical procedure which involves a skin incision must be aggressively treated by peri-operative protocols designed to deliver optimum pain relief. Examples of surgically induced pain are incisional pain or deep-wound pain associated with specific procedures. There are now well-recognised cancer pain syndromes which can be relieved by surgery in the palliative setting but also can be induced or exacerbated by inappropriate or badly judged surgery. Finally, patients presenting with advanced disease (majority in the UK and Ireland) or with local or systemic recurrent disease have pain involvement which is characteristic of their clinical presentation but must be addressed effectively.

Surgical principles for the cancer surgeon

There is a growing recognition among those who are full-time cancer surgeons that certain guiding principles apply to cancer surgery and within these principles many of the iatrogenic and treatment-related cancer pain syndromes can be minimised. These principles are encapsulated in guidelines issued from cancer centres in the USA and include:

- First resection offers the best opportunity for cure.

- Radiotherapy will not improve an inadequate surgical procedure.

- Local tumour recurrence does not always indicate systemic disease.

- Timing of surgical intervention for pain is important.

First resection

First resections are the optimum opportunity for gaining a cure where surgery is the main stay of treatment. Recent advances in radical resectional techniques such as for gastric cancer and total mesorectal excision for rectal cancer enhance local control rates on the one hand, but may potentially increase the risk of physician-induced chronic pain on the other. Thus, where possible, careful pre-operative and intra-operative balancing of the benefits of these curative procedures versus the risks of chronic pain should be undertaken. Much is gained by the use of gold standard staging techniques, where possible. For example, the employment of endoscopic ultrasound which is now known to be the optimum technique for the staging of oesophageal and gastric cancer is essential. This technique is not widely available in the UK and Ireland and thus many patients with advanced cancer (which is primarily surgically incurable) are still receiving treatment which includes the 'look and see' laparotomy. This invariably results in a trial dissection, mainly because the surgeon having come so far is reluctant to 'give up'. Of course palliative resectional procedures may be indicated, such as the resection of advanced gastric cancer where obstruction or bleeding is a problem, but the risk of inducing pain of intractable nature in patients with limited life expectancy must be a primary consideration.

Radiotherapy

Radiotherapy will not improve inadequate surgical excision. While there are situations, such as with rectal cancer, where radiotherapy will improve local control when microscopic involvement of resection margins is noted, there is little benefit of cure, palliation or pain control in giving radiotherapy when macroscopic gross malignant disease exists at the resection margins. Thus a procedure undertaken for the palliative control of cancer pain will be most effective if all gross disease is removed. Simple palliative debulking in many instances is totally inadequate for control of local symptoms because the rapid regrowth of residual tumour will cause a return of pain.

Local recurrence

While local recurrence of tumour is alarming following attempted curative surgery, it must not always be assumed that it indicates systemic disease. Obvious examples are local recurrence of sarcoma and rectal cancers, which tend to behave in this fashion. Some of these patients can be cured following repeat excision and thus careful staging and assessment are required. Thought must be given in these selected instances to further curative resection rather than a less aggressive approach aimed at palliation for pain.

Timing of surgery

The timing of surgical intervention for the relief of cancer pain is paramount. The responsibility of the cancer surgeon must now include an understanding of the biology and natural history of tumours, including an awareness of the likelihood of any invasiveness and the pattern of metastatic disease. When evaluated, these factors may allow the surgeon to consider prospective palliation. This approach could enhance the effectiveness of surgical pain control by undertaking treatment before onset of symptoms. The obvious example is the stabilisation of long bone fractures when fracture is likely. This situation is unlike that of the patient with recurrent intra-abdominal metastatic colorectal cancer whose obstruction may occur at multiple unpredictable levels in the gastrointestinal tract. Prophylatic bypass may only serve to disrupt the patient's quality of life.

Bone involvement

Bone involvement is the third commonest site for metastatic disease, following liver and lung, resulting in a number of complications which include pain, imminent or complete pathological fracture, spinal instability, neurological complications and hypercalcaemia. The exact incidence of bone metastases is uncertain, but in the presence of metastatic disease, bone is involved in 60–84 per cent of cases (Mercadante 1997). In some 85 per cent of cases, the primary lesion arises from either breast, or prostate, or lung (Nielsen *et al.* 1991).

Bone pain

Pain due to bone metastases is the most common cause of cancer-related pain. The exact mechanisms by which metastatic bone disease produces pain are not fully understood, but the release of chemical mediators due to tissue injury, microfractures, nerve root infiltration and compression of nerves due to vertebral collapse are all possible contributing factors in the development of pain due to a malignant bone deposit (Mercadante 1997).

Treatment of bone disease

In the management of malignant bone pain it is important to establish an accurate diagnosis of the cause of the pain and extent of bone involvement. However, the impact on quality of life, and how appropriate management could influence early return to mobility with improvement in quality of life are also of paramount importance. Accurate diagnosis will require good clinical skills with open communication between patient and clinician, the appropriate use of imaging modalities and subsequently a multi-disciplinary approach which results in a comprehensive assessment of the patient, including extent of disease and medical and psychosocial status.

Pathological fractures are associated with the acute onset of bone pain, usually following minor trauma with a low energy injury. Eight to thirty per cent of patients with bone metastases go on to develop pathological fractures, most commonly from carcinoma of the breast. The most common site affected is the proximal femur, although the humerus, vertebrae and pelvis may also be affected (Paterson *et al.* 1991). It is important that the pathological nature of the fracture is identified so that urgent referral to a dedicated orthopaedic surgeon with an interest in malignant bone disease can be made, as the immediate management of pathological fractures differs from that of simple trauma.

The management of painful bone metastases is determined by a multi-disciplinary approach and tailored to suit the individual requirements of the patient. This will involve the use of analgesics following the WHO analgesic ladder (WHO 1996), bisphosphonates to reduce osteoclastic activity and inhibit bone resorption – being mindful of bisphosphonates efficacy in primary diseases, such as myeloma, prostate and breast, with little evidence that they are effective in others – local or wide-field radiotherapy, chemotherapy, hormonal manipulation and surgical intervention. The role of radioisotopes and invasive anaesthetic techniques of neural blockade is not yet clearly defined and may be used to complement other treatment options. Physiotherapy and occupational therapy should be used as part of an overall management plan, and psychosocial support must also be available. The role and evidence for surgery is discussed here.

Surgery for bone disease

The primary aims of surgical intervention are to relieve pain, treat impending or complete pathological fractures, restore function and mobility, in particular where a weight-bearing bone is affected, prevent neurological compromise and possibly prolong survival. The potential benefits of surgery must be balanced against the predicted survival of the patient, and while in many cases of pathological fracture surgery is necessary, in rapidly terminal disease, careful consideration must be given to any surgical intervention (Sabo *et al.* 1998). However, fixation of a pathological fracture in those patients expected to survive only several weeks may still be indicated to relieve pain and allow easier nursing care thus enhancing remaining quality of life (Harrington 1988).

Overall, survival of patients with malignant bone disease has increased in recent years for a number of reasons. Oncological advances in the use of radiotherapy, chemotherapy, hormonal manipulation, etc. are combined with improved orthopaedic intervention, resulting in a multi-disciplinary, multi-modal approach and greater life expectancy. Significant surgical advances include better techniques of fixation, the use of methylmethacrylate bone cement, the development of improved prosthetic implants and, in the last few years, the increasing use of endoprosthesis allowing reconstruction and limb salvage after metastasis resection (Sabo *et al.* 1998). These advances are applicable to the management of lesions in both the long bones and the axial skeleton, and should result in a greater number of patients having specialist orthopaedic assessment and being offered surgery.

Where actual pathological fracture has occurred in a weight-bearing bone, operative fixation should be undertaken, where possible, prior to adjuvant radiotherapy (Hoskin 1995). The indications for prophylactic surgery to prevent pathological fracture and treat painful lesions are less well defined. Where the presence of a tumour results in destruction of 50 per cent or more of the cortex, pathological fracture is considered imminent and prophylactic fixation is indicated (Fidler 1981). Furthermore, in the proximal femur, an avulsion of the lesser trochanter indicates high likelihood of pathological pretrochanteric femoral fracture (Bertin 1984).

Where localised limb pain exacerbated by weight-bearing occurs and X-ray or CT scanning does not show greater than 50 per cent cortical loss, then local irradiation may be indicated (British Association of Surgical Oncology Guidelines 1999). If the pain persists following radiotherapy, it can be assumed that microfractures are present which will progress to complete fracture unless surgery is undertaken (Harrington, 1988).

A more accurate method of prediction of risk of pathological fracture has been proposed by Mirels (1989). This is based on an assessment of 78 cases where a score is given depending on site, size, radiographic appearance of a lesion and associated pain intensity. This can assist in management, where risk of fracture is predicted as low (<5 per cent), intermediate (c. 15 per cent) or high (greater than 20 per cent) (fixation should be carried out.)

When it is decided that surgery is required, the choice of procedure will depend on the site affected. However, three general principles can be applied: the procedure should provide immediate stabilisation of the fracture site, the fixation and implant used should be considered permanent aiming for a single procedure to last the patient's lifetime and, finally, the assumption is made that fracture healing and bony union will not necessarily occur (British Association of British Oncology Guidelines, 1999). With this in mind, rigid fixation augmented by the use of methylmethacrylate cement particularly in the presence of significant cortical defects will satisfy these requirements. The type of internal fixation device to be used will be determined largely by the site affected.

Lower limb

In the lower limb the stresses arising from weight-bearing require secure fixation such as a cemented intramedullary nail for diaphyseal lesions, prosthetic replacement for fractures around the femoral neck (either total arthroplasty or hemi-arthroplasty). These can be done with or without the use of long-term implants to reduce the incidence of periprosthetic fracture or endoprosthesis in limb salvage and reconstruction. It is important to note that stability provided by the fixation device is enhanced by the use of bone cement, which, if used to fill tumour defects and the medullary canal around the implant, will greatly reduce the incidence of implant failure (Harrington 1988).

Upper limb

Metastatic bone deposits are less common in the upper limb, but it is the humerus which is most often is affected and most often requires surgery. Percutaneous intramedullary rod fixation may be used where there is minimal bony destruction, or more rigid fixation with tumour resection augmented by cement in the presence of extensive tumour lysis. Prosthetic joint replacements may be used around the shoulder or elbow, plate and screw fixation may be used where cortical loss is not excessive, as in the case of impending pathological fracture. Unlike the lower limb the non-weight-bearing nature of this bone alters the nature of the type of fixator required and often external methods which may include wire cages are employed.

Spine

In the case of painful spinal metastases, either radiotherapy alone or surgical stabilisation with adjuvant radiotherapy can be offered. Destruction of more than 50 per cent of the vertebral body indicates imminent fracture (De Wald *et al.* 1985), while actual fracture causes vertebral collapse leading to neurological sequelae with compression of nerve roots or spinal cord compression, which is an oncological emergency. While the development of spinal cord compression may require surgical decompression and stabilisation, prophylactic surgery can prevent neurological complications as well as reducing pain and improving ambulation.

Modern surgical techniques of stabilisation have improved in recent years, with tumour resection and spinal stabilisation above and below the resection either by anterior or posterior approach more widely carried out, although the exact criterion for intervention remains controversial. Adjuvant radiotherapy should be given following surgery if and when the wound has healed to reduce residual tumour. The methylmethacrylate cement is not affected by radiation in therapeutic doses, nor does the presence of cement or an implant alter the efficacy of radiotherapy (Harrington 1988).

There is evidence that quality of life is improved for patients having spinal surgery for vertebral metastases, in particular for those with breast cancer metastases. With the use of posterior stabilisation pain is alleviated invariably in 100 per cent with a significant number gaining relief of neurological compromise. The majority derive performance status enhancement. Mobilisation occurs on average by the fourth post-operative day and hospital discharge by the fourteenth day (Okuyama *et al.* 1999). Similarly patients with rectal cancer, breast cancer, melanoma and sarcoma appear to do well with improved quality of life and relief of intractable pain. These patients underwent transthoracic vertebrectomy, decompression, reconstruction with methylmethacrylate and anterior fixation with locking plate and screw. The majority had restoration of ambulation and control of pain thus achieving the primary objective of treatment (Gokaslan *et al.* 1998).

In conclusion, the management of malignant bone pain must be carried out bearing in mind the benefits of orthopaedic intervention or at the very least, specialist referral for consideration for surgery. This is facilitated by a multi-disciplinary approach and case conferences at which the orthopaedic surgeon should have a more definitive role allowing better risk benefits analysis where patients ultimately receive a more realistic appraisal of their situation. There is a need for more randomised controlled trials in the face of evolving techniques to compare therapeutic modalities and assess outcome. Thus patients suffering bone pain due to cancer can receive optimal treatment and be offered the opportunity for improved quality of life.

Newer techniques

There are now a range and choice of pain-reducing techniques which could be employed by the cancer surgeon in the management of cancer pain. For example, transanal endoscopic microsurgery (TEM), which is a minimally invasive technique used to resect rectal lesions by introducing specialist equipment into the inflated rectum via the transanal route. Advantages include mainly the palliation of pain associated with larger infiltrating or obstructing rectal carcinomas in the patient who has a very guarded prognosis or those at high risk for more aggressive transabdominal approaches.

An obvious advantage is the ability to perform repeated procedures for local control of bleeding or painful lesions in very unfit patients. Epidural anaesthesia can be employed for this innovative surgery. Although anaesthesia is needed, this approach can successfully achieve treatment goals in most selected patients (Turler *et al.* 1997). The biggest risk is intra-operative perforation which is likely to occur only in those patients with higher rectal lesions of considerable size and again the employment of repeated procedures over a period of days can reduce the risk. Attention to the curative management of locally advanced rectal cancer also plays a significant role in the overall management of painful primary or recurrent disease. The careful selection of radiotherapy as a neo-adjuvant treatment can reduce local recurrence rates. Accumulating evidence suggests that those with T3 disease or with nodal disease derive a benefit from carefully delivered pre-operative radiotherapy. Evidence suggests that enhancement of disease-free survival can be attained. This will reduce the incidence of postoperative pain and that associated with locally recurrent disease.

However, there appears to be little evidence that post-operative radiotherapy will reduce local recurrence rates and thus the attendant pain (Arnaud *et al.* 1997).

Surgical denervation techniques such as presacral neurectomy for the prophylatic management of pain following resection of uterus, cervix or vagina have been suggested as part of the primary procedure. However, the high rate of complications such as development or worsening of constipation and urinary urgency suggest that more could be lost than gained.

Laparoscopic uterine nerve ablation (LUNA) is a similar approach which employs minimally invasive surgery for the management of pelvic pain. LUNA is often not useful because the pain which requires active management is post-operative thus the operative fields have been disturbed and with development of adhesions minimally invasive techniques are often contraindicated. However, with the growing evidence that minimally invasive techniques may play an increasing role in the management of malignant pelvic and intra-abdominal conditions these techniques should be refined and could play a significant role in the management of cancer pain. There are currently no published randomised trials to support the role of the above techniques in cancer pain management.

Minimally invasive surgery has also been employed to assist in the management of intractable pain associated with coeliac plexus infiltration or damage at surgery. This innovative approach utilises the knowledge that splanchnic nerve outflow arises in the thorax and by introducing thoracoscopes and identifying the tracts in the chest cavity successful nerve ablation can be achieved. This thoracic approach is a minimal surgical insult for the patient and early anecdotal results suggest that effective and long-lasting pain relief can be achieved.

The above techniques describe newer minimally invasive approaches to the surgical management of cancer pain. The advantages for the patient are obvious. The surgical community now has the ability to intervene in a minimally invasive way in both the abdominal and thoracic cavities. With new innovations more aggressive developmental work can be undertaken by interested surgeons in an effort to further reduce problematic pain in cancer patients.

Neuroablative approaches

Many of the more aggressive neuroablative techniques previously used in the management of cancer pain were considered last ditch attempts to relieve intractable pain in patients with rapidly terminal illness. Procedures such as cordotomy, nerve root rhizotomy, pituitary ablation and neurolysis of primary afferent nerves or ganglia did produce pain relief either generally or regionally. No randomised data exist mainly due to the rapidly terminal nature of the illnesses involved. At the present time, many of the treatment objectives of these procedures can now be achieved by regional anaesthetic techniques or the employment of strategically placed needles and delivery of radiofrequencies. These newer approaches, subject to the provision of evidence, may replace surgical approaches to the central and peripheral nervous systems.

Conclusion

The role of surgery in cancer pain control is changing in emphasis. Control of bone pain by prophylactic pinning of long bones or the decompression of the collapsing spine will assume a greater significance. New cements and less invasive approaches mean easier recovery and rehabilitation for the cancer patient. The development of new minimally invasive approaches or the multi-disciplinary management of patients with cancer pain will bring a greater efficacy to pain relief. Finally, the adoption and adherence to strict operative principles by the cancer surgical community can also bring much needed control to chronic post-surgical cancer pain.

References

Arnaud JP, Nordlinger B, Bosset JF, Boes GH, Sahmoud T, Schlag PM & Pene F (1997). Radical surgery and postoperative radiotherapy as combined treatment in rectal cancer. Final results of a phase III study of the European Organisation for Research and Treatment of Cancer. *Br J Surg* **84**, 352–7.

Bertin KC *et al.* (1984). Metastatic malignant disease: isolated fracture of the greater trochanter in adults. *J Bone Joint Surg* **66**A, 770.

British Association of Surgical Oncology Guidelines (1999). The management of metastatic bone disease in the United Kingdom. The Breast Specialty Group of the British Association of Surgical Oncology. *Eur J Surg Oncol* **25**, 3–23.

DeWald RL, Bridwell KH, Prodromas C & Roots MF (1985). Reconstructive surgery as palliation for metastatic malignancy spine. *Spine* **10**, 21.

Fidler MW (1981). Incidence of fracture through metastases in long bones. *Acta Orthop Scan* **52**, 623–7.

Gokaslan ZL, York JE, Walsh GL, Mc Cutcheon IE, Lang FF, Putnam JB Jr, Wildrick DM, Swisher SG, Abi Said D & Sawaya R (1998). Transthoracic vertebrectomy for metastatic spinal tumours. *J Neurosurg* **89**, 599–609.

Harrington KD (1988). Orthopaedic management of metastatic bone disease. The W Mosby Company, St Louis, USA.

Hoskin PJ (1995). Radiotherapy in the management of bone pain disease. *Clin Orthopaed Res* **312**, 105–19.

Mercadante S (1997). Malignant bone pain: pathophysiology and treatment. *Pain* **69**, 1–18.

Mirels H (1989). Metastatic disease in long bones. A proposed scoring system for diagnosing impending pathological fracture. *Clin Orthop Rel Res* **249**, 256–64.

Nielsen OS, Munro AJ & Tannock IF (1991). Bone metastates : pathophysiology and management policy. *J. Clin. Oncol.* **9**, 509–24,

Okuyama T, Korenaga D, Tamura S, Maekawa S, Kurose S, Ikeda T & Sugimachi K (1999). Quality of life following surgery for vertebral metastases from breast cancer. *J Surg Oncol* **70**, 60–3.

Paterson AHG, Ernst DS, Powles TJ, Ashley S, Mc Closkey EV & Kanis JA (1991). Treatment of skeletal disease in breast cancer with clodronate. *Bone* **12**(Suppl.1), S25–30.

Sabo D & Bernd L (1998). Surgical management of skeletal metastases of the extremities. *Orthopade* **27**(S), 274–81.

Turler A, Schafer H & Pichlmaier H (1997). Role of transanal endoscopic microsurgery in the palliative treatment of rectal cancer. *Scand J Gastroenterol* **32**, 58–61.

World Health Organization (1996). Cancer pain relief: with a guide to opioid availability (2nd edn. WHO, Geneva.

Chapter 10

The management of cancer pain in primary care

Stephen Barclay

Introduction

Caring for dying patients at home has long been a central part of the roles of general practitioners (GPs) and district nurses (DNs). This chapter has the following aims:

- to review some of the literature concerning pain control in primary care;
- to summarise some of the research that the Cambridge University Health Services Research Group has undertaken, examining palliative care in primary care;
- to make some recommendations for change.

Figure 10.1 summarises the national data for the place of death of cancer patients. Forty-eight per cent of cancer deaths occur in hospital, and 13 per cent in voluntary hospices. (Currently, the Office for National Statistics only codes deaths in voluntary hospices as hospice deaths: NHS hospice deaths are coded as occurring in NHS hospitals). The remainder of cancer deaths occur under the care of the primary health care team (PHCT): 26 per cent at home, 7 per cent in nursing homes, 4 per cent in residential homes, and 2 per cent in 'other places' (for cancer patients this largely indicates death while staying with relatives). Thus in total, 39 per cent of cancer deaths occur under the care of the PHCT.

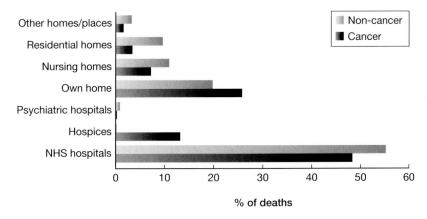

Figure 10.1 Place of death, England and Wales (1995)

But the data for place of death do not tell the whole story. A seminal review article has pointed out that there are two paradoxes concerning place of death (Thorpe 1993). First, that although 'most terminally ill cancer patients would prefer to remain at home, most die in institutions'. It could be added from the literature that most of the lay carers of cancer patients would prefer that death occurred at home (Addington-Hall 1991), and that there is some evidence that this preference for home death declines as illness progresses (Hinton 1994).

Thorpe also noted a second paradox that although 'most of the final year of life is spent at home, most people are admitted to die'. Two studies of nationally representative samples of deaths confirmed that the majority of the last 12 months of life is spent at home, for both cancer and non-cancer patients (Cartwright 1991). Primary care is thus central to palliative and terminal care: most patients would prefer to remain at home, most of their carers would prefer that they remain at home, and most of the last year of life is spent at home under the care of the GP and district nurse.

This key role has long been recognised in national policy documents, such as the report *The Principles and Provision of Palliative Care* (Anon 1992). This stated that 'The Primary Care Team already provide, and will continue to provide, the mainstay of support to patients and families facing terminal illness, even when the act of dying may take place in hospital'.

The control of cancer pain in primary care

Since primary care is central in the provision of palliative and terminal care, it is important to examine how well controlled cancer pain is in this setting. Before doing so, a note of caution needs to be sounded. Being a good generalist is as difficult as being a good specialist: indeed, it is arguably harder. Some specialists, however, seem to gain a degree of satisfaction from pointing out the poor knowledge that their generalist colleagues have in their particular field of expertise. It is hoped that this does not pertain in palliative care, but rather that there is a real partnership between generalist and specialist. Such a relationship is a central thesis of this chapter.

One of the earliest studies was undertaken more than twenty years ago in South London (Parkes 1978). Carers were interviewed approximately one year after the patient's death, and asked to report whether their loved one had experienced 'severe and mostly continuous pain during their final illness'. Six per cent indicated that this was so in what was loosely labelled the 'pre-terminal phase' and 28 per cent in what was loosely labelled the 'terminal phase'; these figures relate to patients cared for at home, largely under the care of the GP and the district nurse (Table 10.1). There was no such increase among those cared for on general hospital wards, and St Christopher's Hospice appeared to be particularly effective in obtaining good pain control in the terminal phase.

Herd (1990) more recently reported a study of terminal care in West Cumbria. Bereaved carers were interviewed six to eight weeks after the patient's death, and

Table 10.1 Proportions of patients with 'severe and mostly continuous pain'

	Home care (%) (n=65)	Hospital care (%) (n=100)	St Christopher's Hospice (%) (n=44)
'Pre-terminal phase'	6	20	36
'Terminal phase'	28	19	8

Source: Parkes (1978)

asked about the presence of symptoms within a loose time period labelled 'terminal care'. (This was simply defined as the period from when care moved from curative to palliative, up to the time of death). During their 'terminal care', it was reported that 69 per cent of 93 patients had experienced some pain, and that for 31 per cent of these 93 patients, the pain had at times been uncontrolled (Table 10.2).

A further study undertaken in Inner London interviewed bereaved carers some eight weeks after the patient's death from cancer (Addington-Hall 1991). Most of these deaths occurred in hospital and not at home: carers were asked questions concerning symptoms in the patient's last week of life. Fifty-seven per cent had experienced pain some time in the last week of life, and for 66 per cent of those, the pain had been severe or very severe (Table 10.3). However, it was reported that analgesia had helped in 80 per cent of patients.

A study of cancer deaths in the Pontefract health district interviewed lay carers six months after the patient's death, enquiring about the presence and severity of symptoms from the time of diagnosis of cancer to the time of death (Sykes *et al.* 1992). Thirty-three per cent were reported to have experienced poor pain control during this period (Table 10.4).

Table 10.2 Patients' symptoms as reported by lay carers (n=93)

	% with problem	% with problem uncontrolled
Loss of appetite	75	74
Weakness	71	69
Pain	69	31
Nausea and vomiting	40	32
Constipation	34	26
Dyspnoea	34	30

Source: Herd (1990)

Table 10.3 Symptoms experienced by patients in the last week of life (n=75–78)

	Patients with symptom	% of those with symptom for whom severe/very severe	% of those with symptom who received treatment which helped
Loss of appetite	78	82	4
Breathlessness	64	51	43
Constipation	64	75	69
Pain	57	66	80
Insomnia	57	51	33
Depression	54	49	10

Source: Addington-Hall *et al.* (1991)

Table 10.4 Carers' recall of symptom control (n=136)

	Patients with symptom poorly controlled (%)
Pain	33
Anorexia	29
Nausea/vomiting	26
Constipation	18
Dyspnoea/cough	13

Source: Sykes *et al.* (1992)

A study in the Devon area looked at cancer deaths, interviewing lay carers some two-to-four months after death, asking them to report the presence and severity of symptoms in the patient's last four weeks of life (Jones *et al.* 1993). All of the deaths occurred at home, the majority of care having been provided by GPs and district nurses, with an input from specialist nurses in a few cases only. Of the 207 patients in the study, 70 per cent had experienced pain in the last four weeks of life, 46 per cent very good pain relief, 20 per cent moderate pain relief, and 4 per cent no relief of their pain (8 of the 207 patients) (Table 10.5).

The authors claim that their study gives evidence of improvement in pain control in the community, highlighting the figure of only 3.9 per cent of patients that obtained no pain relief. It is unclear whether the evidence presented supports such a claim. First, 24.2 per cent were reported to have received moderate or no relief of pain. Second, the study was undertaken in Devon, one of Britain's counties with perhaps a higher standard of primary care than the national average.

Table 10.5 Symptoms in terminally ill cancer patients at home (n=207)

	Patients with symptoms (%)	Very good relief (%)	Moderate relief (%)	No relief (%)
Weakness	72.0	1.0	19.3	51.7
Pain	70.5	46.4	20.3	3.9
Anorexia	69.6	0.0	22.2	47.3
Weight loss	61.8	1.0	22.7	38.2
Constipation	43.5	18.8	20.8	3.9
Insomnia	43.0	7.2	28.0	7.7
Nausea	39.1	10.1	18.8	10.1
Dyspnoea	33.3	9.7	10.1	13.5
Vomiting	32.4	9.2	15.0	9.2

Source: Jones *et al.* (1993)

A seminal paper reported data from two studies of nationally representative samples of deaths from the years 1969 and 1987 (Cartwright 1991). Lay carers were interviewed some months after the patient's death; questions related to care in the whole of the last year of life. For cancer deaths, pain was reported to have been experienced by 87 per cent of patients in 1969, and 84 per cent of patients in 1987, a non-significant fall (Table 10.6). However, for non-cancer deaths, pain had risen significantly from 58 per cent in 1969 to 67 per cent in 1987, and it was the non-cancer deaths that were responsible for the significant overall rise in pain prevalence in the last year of life.

A further paper from a study of a nationally representative sample of deaths reported on deaths from cancer only (Addington-Hall & McCarthy 1995). The study interviewed bereaved carers approximately ten months after the patient's death, asking about their experience during the last year of life of their loved ones. As is true of cancer deaths nationally, most of these cancer deaths occurred in hospital, but most of the last year of life was spent at home under the care of the GP and district nurse. It was reported that 88 per cent of patients had experienced pain some time in the last year of life, and 66 per cent experienced pain some time in the last week of life: for 61 per cent pain was reported to have been very distressing (Table 10.7). Table 10.8 summarises the data concerning pain relief obtained, as reported by the bereaved lay carers.

Table 10.9 summaries the literature described in this chapter, which is not an exhaustive nor a systematic review. The studies come from many areas of the country: the time period assessed ranges very widely from a more loosely defined terminal or pre-terminal period to a more tightly defined period of the last week, last four weeks, or last 12 months. The categories describing poor pain control also vary widely between the studies, making any meta-analysis difficult.

Table 10.6 Symptoms reported by lay carers (%)

	Cancer deaths		Other deaths		All deaths	
	1969 *(n=215)*	*1987* *(n=168)*	*1969* *(n=570)*	*1987* *(n=471)*	*1969* *(n=785)*	*1987* *(n=639)*
Pain	87	84	58	67†	66	72†
Trouble with breathing	47	47	44	49	45	49
Vomiting, feeling sick	54	51	21	27†	30	33
Sleeplessness	69	51*	41	36	49	40*
Mental confusion	36	33	36	38	36	37
Depression	45	38	31	36	36	36
Loss of appetite	76	71	37	38	48	47
Constipation	42	47	23	32†	28	36†
Bedsores	24	28	13	14	16	18
Loss of bladder control	38	37	29	33	32	34
Loss of bowel control	37	25*	24	22	28	23*
Unpleasant smell	26	19	11	13	15	14

† increase $p<0.05$

* decrease $p<0.05$

Source: Cartwright (1991)

Table 10.7 Respondents' reports of symptoms (%)

	Had symptom some time in:		Symptom was
	last year of life *(n=1,886–2,059)*	*last week of life* *(n=1,625–1,988)*	*very distressing* *(n=1,063–1,704)*
Pain	88	66	61
Loss of appetite	78	71	23
Feeling low/miserable	69	47	52
Constipation	62	41	54
Sleeplessness	60	36	34
Dry mouth/thirst	60	49	30
Vomiting/nausea	59	36	56
Breathlessness	54	44	50

Source: Addington-Hall & McCarthy (1995)

Table 10.8 Pain control as reported by carers

Relief from pain treatment given by:	GPs (n=1,344)	Hospital doctors (n=1,047)
Completely all of the time	14	22
Completely some of the time	39	43
Partially/not at all	47	35

Source: Addington-Hall & McCarthy (1995)

Reasons for poor pain control: palliative care research in Cambridge

Dying is therefore 'often an unpleasant and painful process, and there remain many inadequacies in our services to alleviate the distress and create a comforting and supportive environment for the final event in our lives. Technical skills may have contributed to the prolongation of our lives, but adequate services are needed to ensure that this extension is not sometimes a misery for both patients and their relatives' (Cartwright 1991). Furthermore, 'there is still some way to go before all dying cancer patients receive high quality care ... there is, as yet, no room for complacency about the care of dying cancer patients' (Addington-Hall 1995).

More specifically, referring to terminal care at home, Parkes (1978) commented that 'home can be the best place or the worst place to die'. If this is still true, and the above literature suggests so, why is this? Because GPs do not care? Because GPs are poor doctors? The present author believes that these are not the reasons in the great majority of cases. The question of poor pain control is in itself a researchable question that has been addressed in a number of audit and research projects undertaken by the Cambridge Health Services Research Group.

A postal questionnaire study of a random sample of 450 East Anglian GPs investigated their training and knowledge in palliative care. The first questionnaire in this study asked respondents to recall the training they had received during various stages of their careers in a number of key areas of palliative care (Barclay *et al.* 1997) – see Figure 10.2.

Sixty-eight per cent reported receiving training in pain control as clinical medical students, 64 per cent as junior hospital doctors. These percentages rose to 84 per cent during the single year as a GP trainee, and 92 per cent since becoming GP principals. While there was evidence of an improvement in medical student and junior hospital doctor training over recent years, it is still cause for concern that doctors' training is so poor in the early years, especially if one remembers that most cancer deaths occur in hospital under the care of junior hospital doctors. GPs do need training also – an issue that the Macmillan Facilitator network is seeking to address, as are many specialist palliative care services in their local educational programmes.

Table 10.9 Pain control at home: literature summary

Date	Author	Area	Main place of death	Time-period	Poor pain control (%)
1978	Parkes	S London	GP home care	Pre-terminal	6 severe + mostly continuous
1978	Parkes	S London	GP home care	Terminal	28 severe + mostly continuous
1990	Herd	W Cumbria	Home (+ hospital)	Terminal care	31 uncontrolled
1991	Addington-Hall	Inner London	Hospital (+ home)	Last week	66 severe/very severe
1992	Sykes	Pontefract	Hospital (+ home)	From diagnosis	33 poorly controlled
1993	Jones	Devon	GP home care	Last 4 weeks	24 moderate/no relief
1995	Addington-Hall	National	GP home care	Last year	47 partial no relief

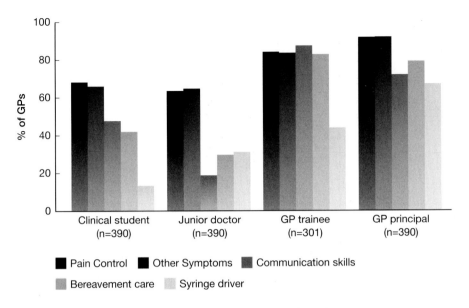

Source: Barclay *et al.* (1997)

Figure 10.2 Reported training in all areas by stage in career (n=390)

The second questionnaire in this study was much more like an examination in format, and designed to test GPs' knowledge in some key pain control issues: a paper containing the data from this questionnaire is shortly to be published. Respondents showed a good understanding of the WHO analgesic ladder, but had some difficulty in the conversion of oral to subcutaneous opioids (see Figure 10.3 overleaf).

Nineteen per cent gave the correct answer of 40 mg, as defined by a Delphi panel of experts and the literature. Twenty-seven per cent gave the possibly correct answer of 41–60 mg, while 16 per cent suggested a significant under-dosage, and another 16 per cent suggested a significant over-dosage. Thirteen per cent would ask for advice, 4 per cent did not know: these responses could arguably be coded as being correct. Six per cent gave no response.

Why are so many GPs finding difficulty with this question? The conversion of morphine to subcutaneous diamorphine is small print for GPs, who rarely set up syringe drivers: perhaps only once or twice a year. If specialists are critical of GPs for not knowing the answers to such questions, perhaps they need to make themselves more freely available to advise their colleagues in primary care over these rare events.

In another of the studies undertaken by the Cambridge group, the views of GPs and district nurses were obtained as to how easy they found to control various symptoms in palliative care at home. GPs reported that they found lack of bowel control the most difficult symptom to control, but saw pain control as the easiest symptom, only 8 per cent rating pain as fairly difficult or very difficult to control.

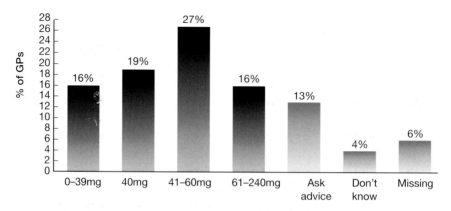

Figure 10.3 Converting MST 60 mg twice a day to 24 hrs dose of diamorphine (n=288)

District nurses had very different views of the difficulty of controlling symptoms, a result which emphasises the importance of teamwork in caring for this patient group. There may be a degree of over-confidence among GPs in their perceptions of the difficulty of controlling pain (see Figure 10.4).

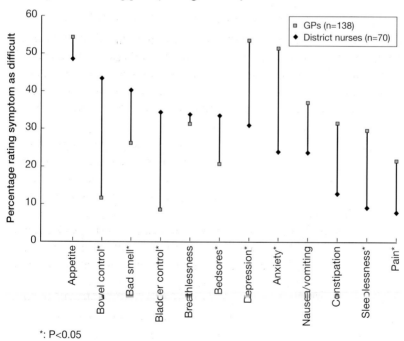

*: P<0.05

Source: Grande *et al.* (1997)

Figure 10.4 Percentage of GPs and district nurses who rated a symptom as very or quite difficult to control

All the literature reviewed at the start of this chapter used a retrospective and proxy methodology. Patients were not asked about their pain themselves: rather, their informal carers were interviewed some months after the person they care for had died. A number of biases come into these data: biases of memory, proxy and bereavement to name but a few. The research group in Cambridge is looking at the methodological and ethical issues of prospective data collection from palliative care patients themselves.

A first step was the development of a prospective proxy methodology, in the development of an audit tool for palliative care in primary care 'CAMPAS' (Rogers *et al.* 1998). In this audit project, GPs and district nurses scored patients' symptoms and needs while providing palliative care for these patients at home.

Figure 10.5 summarises data from 29 terminally ill cancer patients, representing 876 contacts with their GP or district nurse (Rogers 1996). DIS is a *disease impact score*, a modification of the Karnofsky performance scale (Karnofsky *et al.* 1948). When the DIS is 1, 2 or 3, a patient is more mobile and less ill: when the DIS is 4 or 5, the patient is less mobile, and closer to death. The prevalence of severe pain rises from 3 to 14 per cent as death approaches. These figures are cause for concern: they evidence a considerable degree of patient suffering as documented by the GPs and district nurses providing their care.

How would the patients or their informal carers have scored the situation? Our research team is tackling this question in a large scale research study funded by the Department of Health. In this project, we will be asking patients, lay carers, GPs, district nurses, Marie Curie and Macmillan nurses independently to score how severe the patients' pain and other symptoms are, and then compare these different perceptions of the same situation. This study has only completed the pilot phase at the time of writing, so we have no data to present as yet.

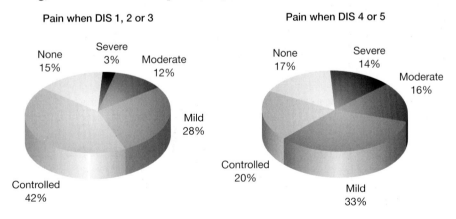

Source: Rogers (1996)

Figure 10.5 Severity of pain as scored by GPs and district nurses (876 contacts with 29 patients)

Changes in primary care

Primary care is changing fast. April 1999 saw the advent of primary care groups that will give GPs and district nurses an increasingly central role in the commissioning of services over coming years. The present author sees this as a real opportunity for specialist palliative care, which in most areas of the country already has strong links with primary care. Our Cambridge research team recently published a study of primary care priorities in palliative care commissioning (Barclay *et al.* 1998), which highlighted the high priority that GPs and district nurses give to the expansion of urgent hospice admission and home care nursing.

The workload in primary care is also changing. With an increasingly elderly population, and the progressive closure of NHS and social security provision for the elderly, recent years have seen a large rise in private residential and nursing homes that are becoming an increasingly important location for palliative and terminal care (see Figure 10.6). In residential homes medical cover is the responsibility of GPs, and nursing care the responsibility of district nurses.

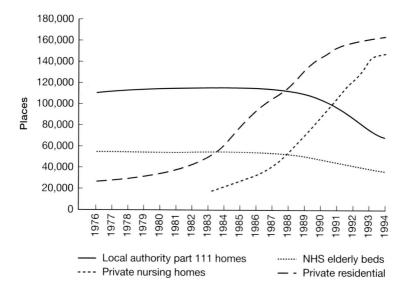

Figure 10.6 Provision of care for the elderly (1976–1994)

Recommendations for change

It is not an option to maintain the *status quo* of palliative care in primary care. There are two ways forward. The first is a stronger response from primary care in terms of symptom control, education and training, personal availability, home nursing services and social care working synergistically with specialist palliative care. The second is a stronger response from specialist palliative care, which effectively represents a take-over of care, with specialist teams assuming 24-hour clinical responsibility. The second model already pertains in a minority of parts of the country where primary care is particularly weak. The present author suggests that this is not the way forward nationally. Most specialists in palliative care would concur with this view.

As long ago as 1986 the medical director of a major specialist home care team wrote that 'there is a danger that specialists may imply that good quality care can only be provided by their experienced team: such a conclusion would progressively undermine the skills of primary and secondary health care colleagues in this area of work. It is never necessary for the specialist team to take over the care of a patient unless that is what the patient and his practitioner want' (Pugsley & Pardoe 1986). While in the short term it may be frustrating for specialist providers to limit their involvement with individual patients in this way, it does allow for the development of mutual trust and respect, and the sharing of specialist skills and knowledge over time. One of the most important attributes of a good GP is the wisdom to know when to refer to specialist services. Calling in specialist help may carry a price for the GP and district nurse, in the loss of control of the patient (Wakefield *et al.* 1993; Brooks 1995), and deskilling as the care is taken over (Field 1998). The present author is aware of a specialist team (a long way from his own city) that is perceived by local GPs to 'take over' patients referred: consequently, few patients are referred by GPs, thus denying them the potential benefits of specialist input and advice. 'It is better to help a colleague with a difficult case than to tell him he is wrong, and that he should make way for the expert' (Pugsley & Pardoe 1986).

If there is to be an improvement in pain control for patients at home, a much stronger response is needed from primary care. GPs and district nurses are the clinicians with long-term relationships with patients and families, and the numbers are simply too great for specialists to take over the care of all patients dying from cancer and non-cancer causes (National Council of Hospices and Specialist Palliative Care Services 1998). Some patients will continue to need multiprofessional specialist care, based in centres and teams of excellence. One of the major and continuing challenges for specialist palliative care is to influence the generalist culture of medical students, student nurses, continuing medical education and practice professional development plans.

Let us work together to make home the best place to die.

References

Addington-Hall J & McCarthy M (1995). Dying from cancer: results of a national population-based investigation. *Palliative Medicine* **9**, 295–305.

Addington-Hall JM *et al.* (1991). Dying from cancer: the views of bereaved family and friends about the experiences of terminally ill patients. *Palliative Medicine* **5**, 207–14.

Anon (1992). The principles and provision of palliative care. Joint Report of the Standing Medical Advisory Committee and Standing Nursing and Midwifery Advisory Committee. HMSO, London.

Barclay SIG, Todd CJ, Grande GE & Lipscombe J (1997). How common is medical training in palliative care? A postal survey of general practitioners. *British Journal of General Practice* **47**, 800–5.

Barclay S, McCabe J, Todd C & Hunt T (1998). Primary care commissioning of services: the differing priorities of general practitioners and district nurses for palliative care services. *British Journal of General Practice* **49**, 181–6.

Brooks D (1995). Palliative care in general practice: should GPs do it at the expense of commoner problems? *BMJ* **311**, 1502–3.

Cartwright A (1991). Changes in life and care in the year before death 1969–1987. *Journal of Public Health Medicine* **13**, 81–7.

Field D (1998). Special, not different: general practitioners' account sof their care of dying people. *Social Science and Medicine* **46**, 1111–20.

Grande GE, Barclay SIG & Todd CJ (1997). Difficulty of symptom control and general practitioners' knowledge of patients' symptoms. *Palliative Medicine* **11**, 399–406.

Herd EB (1990). *British Journal of General Practice* **40**, 248–51.

Hinton J (1994). Can home care maintain an acceptable quality of life for patients with terminal cancer and their relatives? *Palliative Medicine* **8**, 183–96.

Jones R, Hansford J & Fiske J (1993). Death from cancer at home: the carers' perspective. *BMJ* **306**, 249–51.

Karnofsky DA, Abelmann WH, Craver LF & Burchenal JH (1948). The use of nitrogen mustards in the palliative treatment of carcinoma (with particular reference to bronchogenic carcinoma). *Cancer* Nov, 634–56.

National Council of Hospices and Specialist Palliative Care Services (1998). *Reaching out: specialist palliative care for adults with non-malignant diseases*. Occasional paper 14.

Parkes CM (1978). Home or hospital? Terminal care as seen by surviving spouses. *Journal of the Royal College of General Practitioners* **28**, 19–30.

Pugsley R & Pardoe J (1986). The specialist contribution to the care of the terminally ill: support or substitiution? *Journal of the Royal College of General Practitioners* **36**, 47–8.

Rogers M (1996). *Palliative care audit in primary care, report*. Anglia Clinical Audit and Effectiveness Team, University of Cambridge, Cambridge.

Rogers MS, Barclay SIG & Todd CJ (1998). Developing CAMPAS: a palliative care audit for primary health care teams. *British Journal of General Practice* **48**, 1224–7.

Sykes N, Pearson S & Chell S (1992). Quality of care of the terminally ill: the carer's perspective. *Palliative Medicine* **6**, 227–36.

Thorpe G (1993). Enabling more dying people to remain at home. *BMJ* **307**, 915–18.

Wakefield M, Belby J & Ashby M (1993). General practitioners and palliative care. *Palliative Medicine* **7**, 117–26.

Index